YOU WILL FEEL BETTER AND
LOOK BETTER
THAN YOU EVER HAVE BEFORE . . .

Learn how you can eat wisely and well. From family menus to resplendent party fare, these recipes are delicious, varied, ingenious, and inclusive of every possible taste preference and life-style. —from the Introduction by Robert C. Atkins, M.D.

Foods as rich as Oysters Rockefeller . . . quiches . . . blintzes . . . soufflés . . . breads . . . avocado spreads . . .

Such desserts as exotically flavored ice creams and luscious sherbets . . .

Soups . . . meats . . . vegetables . . . and a variety of sumptuous recipes to help you gain energy while controlling weight.

Did you ever dream that dieting could be like this?

DR. ATKINS'
SUPER ENERGY
COOKBOOK

D0441917

SIGNET Books of Special Interest

☐ **THE DIETER'S COMPANION: A Guide to Nutritional Self-Sufficiency by Nikki and David Goldbeck.** Choose the diet that is best suited to you with this essential guide written by two nutrition experts. It includes evaluations of all the well-known diet programs as well as information on designing your own diet according to your weight, health, and food preferences. (#J7401—$1.95)

☐ **THE SOUP-TO-DESSERT HIGH-FIBER COOKBOOK by Betty Wason.** The important new high-fiber, low-calorie diet that adds flavor and good health to every meal you eat! Low-calorie menus, hundreds of delicious recipes, food composition charts and a fiber diet dictionary make this book an absolutely essential kitchen companion for every cook who cares about good health and good eating. (#J7208—$1.95)

☐ **THE LOS ANGELES TIMES NATURAL FOODS COOKBOOK by Jeanne Voltz,** food editor, *Woman's Day* Magazine. Discover the joys of cooking and eating naturally with this book of over 600 savory, simple-to-follow recipes. Whether you are concerned with taste or nutrition, these delicious and healthy recipes—high in fiber content—will delight everyone from the gourmet chef to the dedicated dieter. (#E7710—$2.50)

☐ **LET'S COOK IT RIGHT by Adelle Davis.** Completely revised and updated, this celebrated cookbook is dedicated to good health, good sense and good eating. Contains 400 easy-to-follow, basic recipes, a table of equivalents and an index. (#E7711—$2.50)

☐ **CONSUMER GUIDE®—THE DIET COOKBOOK: Your Guide to Calorie-Wise Gourmet Cooking by Barbara Gibbons and the editors of *Consumer Guide* Magazine.** This book is your key to eating better and gaining less—the only cookbook that lists the calories, protein, carbohydrate, fat and cholesterol content for every recipe and each serving. (#E7265—$2.25)

THE NEW AMERICAN LIBRARY, INC.,
P.O. Box 999, Bergenfield, New Jersey 07621

Please send me the SIGNET BOOKS I have checked above. I am enclosing $_____(check or money order—no currency or C.O.D.'s). Please include the list price plus 35¢ a copy to cover handling and mailing costs. (Prices and numbers are subject to change without notice.)

Name_____

Address_____

City_____State_____Zip Code_____
Allow at least 4 weeks for delivery

DR. ATKINS' SUPER ENERGY COOKBOOK

by
Fran Gare
and
Helen Monica

WITH AN INTRODUCTION BY
Robert C. Atkins, M.D.

A SIGNET BOOK from
NEW AMERICAN LIBRARY
TIMES MIRROR

Published by
THE NEW AMERICAN LIBRARY
OF CANADA LIMITED

NAL books are also available at discounts in bulk quantity for industrial or sales-promotional use. For details, write to Premium Marketing Division, New American Library, Inc., 1301 Avenue of the Americas, New York, New York 10019.

Copyright © 1978 by Fran Gare and Helen Monica

All rights reserved

First Signet Printing, March, 1978

1 2 3 4 5 6 7 8 9

 SIGNET TRADEMARK REG. U.S. PAT. OFF. AND FOREIGN COUNTRIES
REGISTERED TRADEMARK — MARCA REGISTRADA
HECHO EN WINNIPEG, CANADA

SIGNET, SIGNET CLASSICS, MENTOR, PLUME AND
MERIDIAN BOOKS are published in Canada by The New
American Library of Canada Limited, Scarborough, Ontario

PRINTED IN CANADA

COVER PRINTED IN U.S.A.

Acknowledgments

With deep appreciation we would like to thank the following people who gave generously and freely of their time and knowledge to help make this book a reality.

Our attorney, Frank Cohen; the Nutri Plan Staff: Doreen Swan, Kay Goldstein, Margery Korn, Barbara Wright, June Bartley; Helen's husband, Corbett Monica, and our children, David and Marc Gare, Tony, Julie, Nanette, Corvy, and Elena Monica; and those who provided other special services: Dr. José Rodriguez, Mark Adler, Tony De Nicola, and Thelma Welch.

Contents

Foreword

All over America, health is catching. People are becoming more and more aware that they are what they eat.

Americans have always cared a lot about food. Think of it—ours is the only country in the world with an ecumenical harvest feast, Thanksgiving Day. Our national songs proudly glorify "the fruited plains" and "amber waves of grain." We describe ourselves as being as "corny as Kansas in August" or as "American as apple pie." Most of us dearly prize the memory of Grandma's kitchen with its delicious aromas that permeated the whole house.

But we are slowly becoming aware that our foods today are not as nutritious and health-giving as they were in Grandma's day. We are forced to examine our eating habits when the news is filled daily with stories about soil degeneration, pesticide poisoning, pollution contamination, and commercial destruction of food values.

Not so long ago we thought of nutritionists as rather peculiar faddists; after all, who worries about water when water is pure and plentiful? But now we are sitting up and taking notice of what nutritionists have to say.

We are looking for ways to better our diet. We want food that is pure, high in vitamin and mineral content, and free of chemical additives. That is not easy to come by in our modern-day supermarket world of processed foods. Nor is it easy to know what foods are good for us and what foods aren't. And, if we aren't experts ourselves, to whom can we turn for advice?

Advertisers often deceive us. Major food companies have the knowledge but seldom the inclination to help; they still retain a vested interest in the kind of food we no longer want. Our physicians do not help much, since nutrition is at best a three-hour lecture in medical school.

Therefore, the hard job of learning what to eat belongs to the concerned individual. And more and more, that concerned individual represents all of us.

As a society, we are finally becoming nutritionally mature. The rapid growth of health food stores (doing an $8,000,000,000 business yearly) and over-the-counter vitamin sales proves this dramatically. We now have a nutritional Bill of Rights—the federal government's "Truth in Labeling" law—that requires detailed nutritional information on all food products.

We are learning more about nutrition daily. We have found out that nutrition determines not only how you feel and act, but also how you look.

And weight, needless to say, is a major national concern. We are all so concerned about being thin that we are almost compulsively weight-conscious. We want to have it all—sustained youth, super energy, and a glow of health.

The exciting thing is that we *can* have it all with the help of proper eating habits.

Proper eating habits can transform lives. They can mean the difference between intelligence and dullness, a happy person or a grouchy one. With good nutrition comes energy, a glow of the skin, a sparkle to the eye, and a zest for living. It can reshape the body, slow down aging, clear up acne, stop falling hair, and even improve vision.

We want you to be the healthy, happy, glowing people we know you can be. Therefore, we have written this book on food to compliment all of the things Dr. Atkins has told you about energy.

The Super Energy Diet is a diet for a lifetime; we want

to help you improve the quality of your life with good eating habits.

That means introducing you to the health food store with its variety of delicious, fresh, unprocessed, nonchemical foods. We have used many of these foods in our recipes, so if you cannot find an item in your local supermarket, try your health food store.

The grains we use are unprocessed, stone-ground whole grains. They include whole wheat flour, soya flour, rye flour, millet, buckwheat, oatmeal (rolled oats), kasha, couscous, barley, gluten, and wheat germ. All of these should be stored in tightly closed bags and kept in a cool place. Use them quickly, as they contain no preservatives.

Wheat germ and other oil-based foods should be refrigerated after opening. This includes cold-pressed safflower, sesame, wheat germ, peanut and olive oils.

Our favorite quick pick-me-up is a handful of seeds. We use lots of sesame, sunflower, and pumpkin seeds in our recipes. They are high in nutrients and very delicious. Use them generously in soups and salads, with cheese, in main dishes and desserts. Or try toasting them—set your oven to 350°, place the seeds on a cookie sheet and bake for ten minutes. Remove from the oven and season them with oil and sea salt. You won't be able to stop eating them.

Herb teas are another health food specialty. We use several of them in the book, and there are many more. You may enjoy trying some of them. They can help you to relax, stimulate your appetite, act as a diuretic, help prevent disease, or induce sleep. Take your choice of flavors and aromas.

Nor should you overlook the marvelous benefits of eating vegetables and fruits raw. They are a perfect snack and retain all of the vitamins and minerals in their natural form. If you must cook them, steam them. Steamers are available in most houseware stores. Follow the simple directions and the end result will not only be greater flavor and texture but greater health and "economy." (Economy, because when you steam vegetables, the vitamins and minerals are retained and you are getting what you paid for.)

We recommend the use of sugar substitutes because we believe that sugar is far more harmful than the chemicals found in the substitutes. We measure the sugar substitute in packets, one packet equaling two teaspoons of sugar. When used properly, they make satisfying sweet desserts for the weight-loss dieter, and the carbohydrate gram count is amazingly low. This is important to us of course, because our book is about low-carbohydrate cooking—the Dr. Atkins' key to being slim, healthy, and bounding with energy.

We have recipes for three diets. Everyone can use the recipes in Diet 1 (unless they have an allergy to an ingredient in the recipe). Diet 1 is low enough in carbohydrates for the most weight-conscious person.

The recipes in Diet 3 are for people who are at the perfect weight and wish to maintain it. These recipes are higher in carbohydrates and may be used in conjunction with recipes from Diet 1.

The skinnies reading the book will love the delicious, rich recipes of Diet 2. They are the lucky ones who can eat any food in all three diets.

So look for the recipes that pertain to your particular problem.

We have written this book as a gift for all of you who are interested in improving your health. We hope that you enjoy using it as much as we enjoyed preparing it.

HAPPY ENERGY!

FRAN GARE AND HELEN MONICA

INTRODUCTION BY

Robert C. Atkins, M.D.

Why You Need the Super Energy Diet

As a practicing physician, I can assure you that the most common complaint for which a patient walks into a doctor's office is fatigue. And unless that doctor looks for a nutritional cause of the fatigue, chances are he's not going to find the reason.

If he can't find evidence of a sluggish thyroid, anemia, or chronic infection, and if he is still a member of that all-too-prominent segment of the profession which tends to ignore nutrition or takes it for granted, your doctor may conclude that your symptoms are all in your head. Or he may advise you to solve the personal crises in your life.

You know that your symptoms are real. You're not imagining the exhaustion, the inability to concentrate, the strain you've been feeling. Although your doctor might minimize or dismiss their seriousness, as he's trained to view these symptoms in terms of pathology or disease, the effects of chronic fatigue on a person's life are very real and can be serious indeed.

What's more, if you've recently had a checkup and your doctor has tried to reassure you by belittling your complaints, you're likely to feel resigned to your lack of energy and accept it as proof of aging, or "nerves," or the natural consequences of modern life.

Don't accept that conclusion! Even if, like the majority

of the patients I see, you "just plain don't feel well," then you are *not* healthy, your body isn't working efficiently. To conclude that the absence of illness is equivalent to good health is illogical, misleading, and wrong.

Having no energy and a general feeling of malaise may not be a medical mystery; it may be a definite signal of inadequate nutrition. Your body is an intricately calibrated machine which depends on care and maintenance to work efficiently. There is a direct, absolute relationship between what you eat and how you feel. Your health is to a large degree the result of your eating habits: *what* you eat and *how* you eat.

Your tiredness, your lack of energy, even your mood swings will vanish when the treatment is directed to the real cause.

That treatment, more often than not, is a new diet and a new emphasis on nutrional techniques. The diet that will restore your energy and feeling of well-being is the Super Energy Diet.

Even if you feel fine and consider yourself healthy, the Super Energy Diet is important to you. I have seen dramatic improvements in the health and energy of virtually every one of my patients who has used the Super Energy Diet—including those who thought they felt fine to begin with.

If you were to tell me, "I eat a proper, balanced diet already," I'd have to respond that this probably isn't true. Nutritionally oriented doctors and scientists are finding obvious, demonstrable proof that the American diet is inadequate and nutrionally impoverished. Malnutrition has become a major national health catastrophe.

Dr. Roger Williams, considered to be one of the founding fathers of the new science of clinical malnutritional medicine, lists the number one axiom of the science to be, "Everyone has suboptimal nutrition." This is his way of saying that in every case, there is room for improvement.

Does this sound as self-evident to you as it does to me?

Well, it is not self-evident to the leaders of American medicine—the AMA, FDA, and their colleagues. Their opinion is that all the nutritional help we need can be derived from a balanced diet chosen from among the four basic food groups; anything beyond that, they consider to be quackery, hogwash, or even dangerous. In other words, there is no room for improvement in most of us.

Then why do I *see* improvement in all of my patients once I've begun to modify and correct their nutritional patterns?

The decision is yours; you *do* have choices. It's important for you to take responsibility for your own body. I want you to rely on your own sound judgment.

If you suspect that there *is* room for improvement in your energy levels and general feeling of well-being, try the Super Energy Diet. It offers more than freedom from fatigue and chronic exhaustion—it is a way of life, a constant state of dynamic good health.

And let's begin with a clear eye on reason and reality. There's no room in a rational diet plan for miracles, shortcuts, illusions, or tricks. I wish there were some vitamin-laden, energy-packed food that would overcome all our nutritional sins and restore us to the level of energy we were all meant to have.

But, of course, it isn't that easy. The key to personal nutrition and discovering your own source of Super Energy involves a total revision of your diet.

To understand the principles of the Super Energy Diet, you will have to understand these two key words: RESTRUCTURE and REDIRECT. Your entire diet must be completely *restructured* for the purpose of *redirecting* your pathways of energy metabolism.

Let me show you how it works.

First, you must learn about your blood sugar levels. You may be thinking, "I'm sure I have no abnormality in my blood sugar levels; my doctor checked everything and he found nothing wrong. I'm not sick, I'm just tired." Or your reaction might be just the opposite: "I know I have low blood sugar; I have so many symptoms."

Perhaps we should put the matter of low blood sugar aside for a moment to point out that everyone has a level of sugar (as glucose) in his blood, and that it goes through some significant variations in the course of each day, depending on what and when we've eaten, if we've had exercise, what amounts of physical and emotional stress we've endured, and so on.

What's so important about blood sugar? Two things. First, it's a source of fuel for your body, and second, it feeds the brain and nervous system directly. When the blood sugar level drops too low, the brain and nerves can develop signs of starvation; they don't work well. You may notice symptoms of confusion, inability to concentrate, anxiety, irritability, trembling, light-headedness.

Here's how the metabolism of blood sugar works.

The carbohydrates that you eat are converted to *glucose* during the process of digestion. Glucose enters the bloodstream from the small intestine; its presence stimulates the production and release of insulin, a pancreatic hormone whose function is to control blood sugar. Insulin is the agent that causes absorption of glucose into the liver cells, where it is stored as *glycogen*.

Essentially then, the physical equation is

CARBOHYDRATE $\longrightarrow$ GLUCOSE $\longrightarrow$ GLYCOGEN

digestive   insulin
enzymes

But for most of us who have been exposed to a diet in which the quick-acting, refined carbohydrates predominate, that insulin response gets to be somewhat more than enough to process the influx of sugar, and the result is that the glucose level, which rose as it was absorbed into the bloodstream, soon drops to a point *below* where it was before we ate. When this happens, *we are hungry and have less energy after we have eaten than we did before.*

And this rebound effect continues. When the blood sugar level drops significantly, and there is still an abundance of insulin present in the blood, the adrenal glands are stimulated to produce *adrenaline.* Adrenaline blocks insulin activity and causes the *reconversion* of glycogen to glucose, which is then released into the bloodstream until a balance is restored; then it's time to eat, and the whole thing starts again.

This physiologic pattern is *not* caused by insufficient sugar ingestion but by a consistently overreactive insulin response. Hypoglycemia is most accurately described as a metabolic intolerance to sugar (and carbohydrate) and the inability to use it efficiently.

The biochemical yo-yo syndrome I've described as typical of hypoglycemia produces concomitant physical and emotional gyrations. This explains the fluctuations in your energy level and mood and alertness. Furthermore, the adrenaline response presents the unpleasant symptoms you associate with an anxiety attack: rapid pulse rate, trembling, excessive perspiration, apprehension, dizziness, visual disturbances, irregular heart rhythms, fainting spells, and, not infrequently, migraines.

You may recognize some or all of the symptoms I've mentioned and feel convinced that you're suffering from hypoglycemia. Or, if you don't seem to fit into the patterns I've described, you might conclude that you definitely aren't hypoglycemic. Either assumption will be no more than an educated guess, and guesswork is an inappropriate and unsound approach to a medical diagnosis.

There is a simple, direct, scientific procedure to establish the diagnosis of hypoglycemia: the glucose tolerance test (GTT). Its use is the focal point of an intense medical controversy concerning hypoglycemia. Doctors who routinely give glucose tolerance tests say: "I see alot of patients with hypoglycemia"; doctors who don't use the GTT say: "I see none."

My clinical experience with these test results has demonstrated that the vast majority show abnormal blood sugar curves, presenting either a definite diagnosis of hypoglycemia (or diabetes), or enough instability in blood sugar levels to merit dietary changes.

If ever there was a condition that is nutritional in its cause and nutritional in its cure, that condition is hypoglycemia.

Because our levels of energy and mood and mental capacity fluctuate along with our blood sugar levels, the essential question is: Would stabilizing these blood sugar gyrations improve any of the symptoms?

Speaking from the vantage point of a doctor who sees patients at weekly intervals, and has asked that question of thousands of them, I can assure you that the answer in the overwhelming majority is "YES!" Yes, by stabilizing the blood sugar, almost everyone, even those people whose glucose tolerance tests are classified as "normal," will notice improvements in mood and energy.

The secret, if there is a secret, to achieving Super Energy is just that: restructuring the entire diet to achieve equilibrium or stability in the levels of metabolic fuel, of which the most changeable is glucose, the blood sugar.

Here's how it's done.

The Super Energy regimen has two major thrusts of effectiveness. One is based on these dietary restructurings; the other involves the use of vitamin therapy, based on some highly sophisticated biochemical principles, for the purpose of redirecting the metabolic pathways over some presumed areas of blockage.

To understand and apply these principles of vitamin therapy, I must refer you to the rather detailed discussion of vitamins and minerals in my book, *Dr. Atkins' Super Energy Diet*. This present book deals with dietary changes and shows you how your cooking can be developed to create the most healthy, appealing meals with inventive, delicious recipes and nutrition information, with which you'll be able to make a Super Energy Diet a permanent way of life.

The Super Energy Diet

The first premise to bear in mind is that, although there are basic principles of dietary management which do apply to most people, there cannot be a *single* diet that's effective for everyone. We simply do not all respond the same way. How many of you, for example, have noted that, in any group of people, there are some who will gain weight and some who will lose following the same diet? This is a very obvious example of metabolic differences among individuals. The doctor working in the field of nutrition sees the same variability with regard to each and every nutritional factor.

The person who tends to gain weight on random eating is metabolically quite different from one who tends to lose weight. Quite logically, the person who tends to maintain normalcy in his weight has a metabolic response approximately midway between these extremes. Accordingly, to deal with these three general types, three basic dietary regimes must be used in the Super Energy Diet. I've labeled them:

Diet 1 The Super Energy Weight-Losing Diet
Diet 2 The Super Energy Weight-Gaining Diet
Diet 3 The Super Energy Stay-the-Same-Weight Diet

Diet 1 should be familiar to all of you who are not my first-time readers, for it was the diet featured in my first book, *Dr. Atkins' Diet Revolution.*

It is based on the now axiomatic observation that the

single most effective diet for the combined control of energy, mood, *and* overweight in the overweight individual is the diet *lowest* in carbohydrate.

This is true because the overweight person is uniquely resistant to the metabolic problems which carbohydrate-restricted diets pose for the average individual. In fact, the major features of metabolic imbalance which led to his being overweight in the first place are all directed toward making him inordinately efficient at converting his dietary protein and fat into carbohydrate-like metabolites. His body chemistry is extremely keto-resistant. (In other words, he is fat because he has greater difficulty than the average person in breaking down his fat stores so that they can be used as fuel.)

Diet 1 works like this:

The main objective of the tired person who is also overweight is to convert to alternative forms of metabolic fuel those derived from the stores of excess body fat. That way, both the energy problem (due to unstable rate of fuel supply) and the weight problem (due to excessive stores of body fat) can be solved at the same time.

When fat burns, it breaks down into two metabolic fuels: free fatty acids, which can be utilized by muscular tissue, and ketone bodies, which the brain and blood cells can utilize. We can detect the presence of both these fuels, but the ketone bodies are more easily detectable by a simple urine dipstick (called a Ketostik), and thus a person who is burning his fat stores, through any very effective diet, is said to be in *ketosis*.

The basic principle of Diet 1, then, is to achieve this desired burning of the fat stores in the easiest, most expedient and efficient way. If we understand the "picking order" in which the body chooses its fuels, which are alcohol, sugars, starches, fats, and proteins, we can deduce that by eliminating alcohol and carbohydrates (sugars and starches), fat becomes the first of the remaining fuels to serve as the primary fuel source.

And that is what we do. In the pure form of the diet, we eliminate the carbohydrate and alcohol and are left with a diet consisting entirely of protein and fat. This means that meat, eggs, fish, fowl, and cheeses become the mainstay of the diet and that fats and oils can also be permitted. Years of observing dieting patients have shown that some carbohydrate—up to 20 or 30 grams daily in the average person—allows the desired body chemistry to continue in much the same way as it did when no carbohydrates were allowed.

What each Diet 1 dieter must learn is the level of carbohydrate in his own biochemical response which gets him out of ketosis (according to the Ketostik), for this is his own personal Critical Carbohydrate Level. Having made this determination, he then knows how many grams of carbohydrate he can allow himself if he wishes to continue the combined effects of blood sugar control and weight loss.

Diet 1, then, has varying levels. This variance serves to allow for the individualization and tailoring of the diet to match the biochemical responses which are so sorely lacking in most other diet regimens.

Diet 2, is, of necessity, quite different, because the metabolism of the underweight individual is quite different.

The underweight biochemical type has a very inefficient metabolism, and there is much wastage of fuel. Therefore, he can eat great quantities of food without gaining weight. For him, carbohydrates are necessary to prevent even further weight loss.

This poses a very difficult dilemma for the underweight person who is seeking to stabilize his blood sugar. The best way to achieve this result is to make sure that the carbohydrates taken in are not converted into sugar rapidly but rather in the most roundabout way, so that the release of insulin can be gradual and a balance can be maintained—without overshooting the mark. This is done by using starches as they occur in nature, unrefined or processed, which are then broken down by the digestive enzymes and converted from complex carbohydrates into simpler ones.

Therefore, the principles of Diet 2 involve using starchy carbohydrates (but not refined starches, such as flour) which the body can attack slowly—rather than sugars. The other principles of blood sugar regulation involve:

1. Frequent feedings.

2. Spacing of the carbohydrates throughout the day. Both these techniques stabilize the blood sugar by providing a more or less constant intake of metabolic fuel.

3. Avoidance of drugs which affect the insulin or sugar levels directly. Caffeine is an important example of such a drug; alcohol has this rapid effect as well—and must be avoided, or taken in very slowly.

When devising recipes for Diet 2 we have taken care to provide that the carbohydrates are not simple sugars and starches; instead, we use brown rice, whole grains, lentils, vegetables, nuts, and seeds.

Diet 3 falls somewhere in between these two diets, and the foods and recipes that can be utilized in this diet are similar to those for Diet 2 but are still on the low total carbohydrate side. For most people, this means around 60 carbohydrate grams per day.

On Diet 3, you're allowed all the foods on Diet 1, in addition to:

(1) 2 to 3 slices of gluten bread, or one slice of stone-ground wheat bread, or two slices of whole rye flatbread (up to 15 carbohydrate grams per day);

(2) olives, nuts, and seeds (as much as you like, with the exception of chestnuts, water chestnuts, and cashews, which are high in carbohydrates).

After the first two weeks, you may find that you are gaining weight or losing weight—although you've stuck to the diet carefully. The first remedy you should try is using Diet 2 for a while; by eating generously, while in ketosis, you can reverse an unexpected weight gain or return the weight you've lost on Diet 3.

If your weight loss continues on Diet 3, you may need more carbohydrates. Here are two gambits that I have used successfully. One adds a form of simple sugar, fructose, which you can get in tablet or powder form. You can use about 30 carbohydrate grams a day of fructose, and supply the remaining 30-gram allowance with any of the other carbohydrates you like.

The other variation is the addition of whole grains or lentils, plus oats, barley, millet, maize, or brown or wild rice (in the same proportions you used in adding fructose).

Caution: If you are purchasing precooked whole-grain products—cereals, breads—read the labels carefully! "Whole wheat" products frequently contain bleached flour too. The best choice would be to use the many recipes in this book—listed with Diet 3—that use only the grains and lentils you're allowed.

Whether you decide to use fructose or grains as your carbohydrate "booster" is really a matter of your taste preferences and life-style. Which do you prefer/miss more—sweets or starches? Whichever you decide to add, fructose or grains, remember not to change more than one variant at a time, so that you know exactly what is causing the results you get.

As long as your weight is stable, you can keep at this gram level and try all the foods that appeal to you in the Diet 3 recipe section.

Nutritional Villains and Valiants

To change your eating habits, as well as your buying habits, you must be willing to reeducate yourself; you must go farther than a set of maxims of "how-to." You need more than a passing acquaintance with what foods to *avoid*—the most notorious health thieves as well as the more oblique detours from sensible eating that belie their content with appealing packaging and marketing devices. We've all been victims, at one time or another, of that kind of ploy.

To select food intelligently, you must arm yourself with knowledge and steel yourself with righteous discipline!

Energy Thieves

There is no doubt that the single largest fault in the American diet is the consumption of refined carbohydrates. It is reported that 80 percent of the total caloric intake in this country comes from the following deficient foods: white sugar predominantly, white flour, and all the products containing them.

Refined carbohydrates are nutritionally empty, a violation of nature; they offer "purity" at the expense of nutrition.

Refined sugar does the greatest harm in many ways: it is a starvation food because it satisfies your call for food but leaves thousands of hungry cells misbehaving and dying because they don't get the enzymes, proteins, minerals, and vitamins they need (they were removed in the refining process); it is an antinutrient because it uses up B-complex vitamins and essential trace minerals; it can be addicting, setting up the vicious cycle of hypoglycemia, or what's come to be known as "the junk-food syndrome"; it can also be the cause of hyperkinesis in children, or the factor underlying a diagnosis of MBD (minimal brain damage).

The other carbohydrate that is a nutritional villain is "pure" white flour. Here again, refining does the irreversible damage. The highly nourishing germ of the wheat is very rich in oil (wheat-germ oil). This is discarded in the refining process because it becomes rancid quickly, and makes the flour unpalatable. The outer coat, called the bran, is rich in minerals and is also high in the B-complex vitamins. Insects thrive on this, and they find it quickly after it is ground into flour. Therefore, the bran is removed so that flour can have commercial shelf-life and shipping value.

The discarded wheat middlings are rich in essential minerals; some protein values are destroyed in the milling. Milling grains—stripping their nourishment, and then "enriching," which means adding three synthetic vitamins and iron—is both an outrage and an insult to our intelligence. As long as people continue to buy plain white flour, it will be packaged and sold, mislabeled as "food."

NOTE: *The Super Energy Diet holds a unique position in regard to additives: I caution you to avoid all additives except sugar substitute. Because the basic foundation of the Super Energy Diet is the stabilization of blood sugar, we feel that the function of artificial sweeteners is important and necessary in a sugar-free diet. It's pleasant to eat sweet-tasting food occasionally without the dangerous consequences of low blood sugar. The recipes in this book are designed to utilize the non-nutritive sweeteners available at this time.*

High-Energy Foods

We require daily replenishment of all the essential nutrients found in natural, vital foods. There are some that are so rich in nutritional value that they should be routinely incorporated into your diet. They can be likened to high octane gasoline: they deliver more pep and promote a greater output of energy.

SUNFLOWER SEEDS should be a permanent addition to a Super Energy Diet. For victims of hypoglycemia, they are invaluable. They raise the blood sugar naturally, through their protein content. They are one of the best snack foods available: a few sunflower seeds for "the afternoon slump" or to nibble when traveling will give you an energy boost within minutes!

BREWER'S YEAST is one of the best high-energy foods; it is richer in total protein than almost any other food, which means it has exceptional value in promoting weight loss and providing energy. (*Note:* Because it also contains some carbohydrate [3 grams per ounce], it should not be used at the beginning of Diet 1; you must carefully count its carbohydrate grams when you include it in your daily allowance.)

LECITHIN is found in every cell of the body and should be constantly replenished to prevent a deficiency in any of the important body functions. Because lecithin contains phosphorus, it is needed by the brain; it's a natural tranquilizer as well. It can also help to distribute weight more evenly.

If you're concerned with the fat and cholesterol that are important in the Super Energy Diet, take lecithin. It contains choline and inositol, B-complex vitamins that work as cholesterol emulsifiers or dissolvers.

Lecithin is available in three forms: liquid, powder, and granules. It is tasteless, but the liquid is very sticky and somewhat unpleasant to swallow. The recipes in this book use lecithin in powder or granule form.

WHEAT GERM is another excellent natural food. It is the part of the whole grain that is removed in the milling process—the part with the greatest vitamin, mineral, and protein content. Wheat germ has long been an essential ingredient in the diet of athletes—it is invaluable in building energy and fighting fatigue.

SOYBEANS are rich in protein and even higher in calcium and other alkaline minerals than the best meat. The balance of essential amino acids (the amino acids or protein factors that the body can't produce) in soybeans is not the same as that in meats, however, so more grams of this protein are needed to supply them adequately. Considered "the poor man's steak," soybeans can offer even more variety to a high-protein diet.

NUTS are rich sources of protein too, and carry all the essential amino acids. They should be used generously in our diets—eaten unroasted, since heating destroys some of their nutritive value.

SESAME SEEDS contain significant amounts of lecithin, choline, and inositol for healthy blood vessels and strong nerves. When ground, they are an excellent flour-substitute base. (There are many recipes in this book using ground sesame seeds.)

WHOLE GRAINS, such as barley, oats, wheat, kasha, and millet, offer substantial amounts of protein. Millet can be used like any of the seeds—sunflower, sesame, pumpkin—in baking.

SPROUTS are probably the healthiest food on earth. Sprouting seeds offer a fresh, crisp food that compares with meat in nutritional value, fresh fruit in vitamin C, that has no waste, is excellent raw, and can be cooked in a few minutes. You can sprout seeds at home, or buy them already sprouted at health food stores and some supermarkets. They are one of the least expensive sources of natural vitamins you can find.

Of course no single substance will maintain good health, but these natural foods are richer in many nutrients than most. By incorporating them into your diet, you can avoid eating large amounts of less potent foods that merely fill you up. They're a good value financially, because they are full of free vitamins, minerals, and amino acids that would cost much more were you to buy them separately.

Each of these foods is like banking nutritionally. It is a safe assumption that there are many nutrients as yet undiscovered; they're most probably present in foods like these, the sources of so many key nutrients.

This cookbook was written to answer the questions I'm most frequently asked by patients who are beginning the diet. The most compelling (and probably the least verbalized) is: How will I stand it? How can I live with such Spartan resolve all my life—giving up oral gratification for the sake of my health?

The answer is in two parts. First, you won't feel a bit martyred; you need not give up the physical, esthetic, emotional, and sensual pleasures of eating. You'll feel none of the deprivation or boredom that you associate with the wretchedness of dieting. You'll eat butter and cream sauces, bacon and eggs, lobster, vichyssoise, omelets, salad dressings, and even sweet-tasting desserts! *You'll never be hungry!*

The other important point is that this diet life-style will affect your intellect as well as your body: your values will change—learning good nutrition is really behavior modification. My primary goal is to get you to take care of yourself and to teach you how to eat for the rest of your life. Food will become both less important and more important: it will not be a thinly disguised substitute for love, or esteem, or ego gratification (when you like yourself, you no longer need childish ploys or substitutes for respect and affection); furthermore, you'll like food better when you're more aware of its intrinsic value; you'll no longer take it for granted—you'll come to appreciate food in many new ways.

When I give my patients a list of foods for their Super Energy Diet, I usually hear a barrage of puzzled, dismayed questions:

"Cut out all flour?! How?"

"What's lecithin? How do I get it?"

"Eat millet and sprouts and kasha? What are they? How do I cook them?"

This book provides all the answers. You already know what "they" are; the rest of the book will explain where to purchase these foods, in what form to buy them and store them, and, best of all, how to cook irresistible dishes with some ingredients that will be new to you, as well as variations on your long-standing favorites.

Invariably, the patients who leave my office armed with their new diet and a nagging sense of doubt are the ones who return saying, "How did I stand it before I began the diet? I've never felt better in my life!"

I want you to start the Super Energy Diet—and stick to it for the rest of your life. Once you achieve your ideal weight, you'll be able to maintain it permanently on Diet 3, without ever feeling deprived or cheated of good food.

You'll always look your best and function at a constant peak of energy, creativity, efficiency, enthusiasm, and high spirits.

Not only will you favorably impress everyone with whom you come in contact, but you'll find, as well, that *you're* more interested and stimulated by the world.

And what's more, you'll find that your exuberant good health is catching!

Start reading the recipes in the book to learn how you can eat wisely *and* well. From family menus to resplendent party fare, these recipes are delicious, varied, ingenious, and inclusive of every possible taste perference and life-style.

The greatest investment you make in life is in yourself. Start now, with a new beginning of vitality, well-being, and lifelong good health!

NOTE

It is important to us that you not be limited by the diet categories in this book, for many of you will be able to use recipes from all three diets.

For example, those of you on Diet 2 may enjoy not only Diet 2 recipes but can also use Diet 1 and Diet 3 recipes. Those of you on Diet 3 can use any of the Diet 1 recipes as well as any Diet 2 recipes with a low gram count.

The only group of dieters who are limited are those on Diet 1—they can use only Diet 1 recipes until they have graduated to the "Maintenance Diet."

When using the Meal Plans, check the Index and gram counts so you don't overextend your daily carbohydrate gram allowance.

DIET I

MENU PLAN
FOR DIET 1

DAY ONE

Breakfast:

Ham and eggs
   Coffee-Maple Breakfast Protein

Lunch:

Fish Fillets with Scallop Sauce
   Cottage cheese with one tablespoon chopped onion
      Coffee or tea

Dinner:

Chicken India
   One cup greens with Italian Dressing
      Two Coconut Candies

Snack:

One serving Sponge Torte

DAY TWO

Breakfast:

   Two soft-boiled eggs
      One slice Hi-Protein Soya Bread
      One slice Swiss cheese
         Hot Coffee Protein Drink

Lunch:

   Sicilian Fish
      One cup greens with Italian Dressing
         Coffee, tea, or diet soda

Dinner:

   Garlic Soup
      Eggplant Parmigiana
         Coffee or tea

Snack:

   One serving Chocolate Sponge Layer Cake
      Diet soda

DAY THREE

Breakfast:

Two tablespoons cottage cheese on slice of Hi-
Protein Soya Bread
    Coffee or tea

Lunch:

Spicy Cauliflower Soufflé
    Sliced tomato with Creamy Celery Seed Dressing
        Coffee, tea, or diet soda

Dinner:

Fran's Special Pâté
    Baked chicken with Apricot or Peach Glaze
        Lettuce

Snack:

One serving Spice Cake

DAY FOUR

Breakfast:

Cheese omelet
Coffee or tea

Lunch:

Quick Poached Fish Fillets
Assorted greens salad with Tarragon Dressing
Coffee, tea, or diet soda

Dinner:

Clams Casino
Veal Rolls
Two Spice Cookies

Snack:

One serving Light Sponge Cake
Diet soda

DAY FIVE

Breakfast:

Two slices Hi-Protein Bread toasted
Berry Jam
Coffee or tea

Lunch:

Green Onion and Red Caviar Quiche with crust
Coffee, tea, or diet soda

Dinner:

Mrs. Landau's Shrimp Sauté
Zucchini Milano
Melon

Snack:

Assorted hard cheese cubes

DAY SIX

Breakfast:

Two pieces French Toast
with a sprinkle of cinnamon
Two soft-boiled eggs
Coffee or tea

Lunch:

Confetti Mold
Four tablespoons cottage cheese
Coffee, tea, or diet soda

Dinner:

Beef Stroganoff
One cup lettuce with
Parmesan Caesar Dressing

Snack:

Brewer's Yeast Hibiscus Drink

DAY SEVEN

Breakfast:

Creamy Peach Omelet
Cool Lime Mint with Lecithin

Lunch:

Peppered Fish
Spinach Salad with Avocado Dressing
Coffee, tea, or diet soda

Dinner:

Tony's Cream of Chicken
One cup greens with Italian Dressing

Snack:

One piece Almond Coconut Candy
Diet soda

DAY EIGHT

Breakfast:

Two scrambled eggs with Cream Sauce
    Diet soda

Lunch:

Frozen Berry and Nut Salad
    Coffee or tea

Dinner:

Calves Liver in Red Wine
    Broccoli with Sharp Sauce
        Lemon Cake Custard Pudding

Snack:

Marbleized Tea Eggs from China

DAY NINE

Breakfast:

Boursin and Lecithin Omelet
Diet soda, coffee, or tea

Lunch:

Chicken and Egg Loaf
½ cup lettuce with two tablespoons
Sour Cream or Mayonnaise Dressing
Coffee or tea

Dinner:

Cucumber Soup
Moussaka

Snack:

One Spice Cookie
Diet soda

DAY TEN

Breakfast:

Alfalfa and Cheddar Cheese Omelet
Diet soda, coffee, or tea

Lunch:

Fish Soufflé
One cup greens with Italian Dressing
Coffee or tea

Dinner:

Swiss Chicken
Cranberry Frost

Snack:

One piece Coconut Candy
Diet soda

DAY ELEVEN

Breakfast:

Reuben Omelet
Coffee or tea

Lunch:

New England Fish Chowder
Ham sandwich with Hi-Protein Bread
Coffee or tea

Dinner:

Steak au Poivre
Peanut Butter Ice Cream

Snack:

One serving cold chicken
with one tablespoon Thousand Island Dressing
Diet soda

DAY TWELVE

Breakfast:

   Bacon and eggs
      Mocha Breakfast Drink

Lunch:

   Roquefort Quiche
      U.S. Hamburger
         Coffee or tea

Dinner:

   Shrimp and Scallops Mark
      ½ cup boiled cauliflower
         One serving Confetti Mold

Snack:

   One cup diet soda

DAY THIRTEEN

Breakfast:

   Blintz Omelet
     Diet soda, coffee, or tea

Lunch:

   Crunchy Seafood Salad
     Black Cow

Dinner:

   Meat Loaf Supreme
     Seasoned Spinach
       Almond Custard

Snack:

   ¼ cup melon balls

DAY FOURTEEN

Breakfast:

Basic Omelet
Bacon
Coffee or tea

Lunch:

Zucchini Parmesan Quiche
Cottage Cheese Dessert Salad
Coffee or tea

Dinner:

Baked Fish with Sour Cream
Mushroom and Celery Sauté
Two Chocolate Peanut Butter Cookies

Snack:

Diet soda

RECIPES
FOR DIET 1

———◆———

Appetizers, Dips, and Fillings

SAVORY SANDWICH FILLINGS

Reuben Filling

1 slice corned beef, finely
    minced
1 slice Swiss cheese, finely
    minced

2 ounces cream cheese
1 tablespoon heavy cream
1 teaspoon prepared mustard

Combine all ingredients. Blend thoroughly.

TOTAL GRAMS 3.5

Nutty Olive Filling

4 stuffed olives, finely
    minced
6 walnut halves, chopped

2 ounces cream cheese
1 teaspoon olive juice

Combine all ingredients. Blend thoroughly.

TOTAL GRAMS 5.8

Salmon Ball

1 cup canned salmon
4 ounces cream cheese
1 teaspoon lemon juice
¼ teaspoon chopped dill
1 tablespoon minced onion
1 tablespoon juice from
    can of salmon

½ teaspoon white horse-
    radish
¼ teaspoon onion salt
¼ cup chopped walnuts
1 tablespoon chopped parsley

Remove skin and bones from salmon meat.

Blend thoroughly with remaining ingredients except nuts and parsley. Shape into a ball. Wrap in aluminum foil and refrigerate for several hours.

Remove foil and roll ball in nuts and parsley.

Makes 6 servings.

2.7 GRAMS PER SERVING

Sardine Dip

1 can skinless and boneless
    sardines, drained
3 hard-boiled eggs, mashed
6 ounces cream cheese,
    mashed
¾ teaspoon lemon juice

½ teaspoon dried parsley
¼ teaspoon dill weed
¼ teaspoon salt
2 tablespoons chopped
    onion

Combine all ingredients in a blender or food processor until smooth.

Makes 6 servings.

1.0 GRAM PER SERVING

Fran's Special Pâté

4 slices bacon (without ni-
trates if possible)
1 pound chicken livers
1 chicken cutlet, pounded
flat
4 teaspoons seasoned salt
2 tablespoons butter
2 tablespoons white wine

½ of an 8-ounce can water
chestnuts
2 hard-boiled eggs
1 Boursin cheese
3 tablespoons sweet basil
3 tablespoons chicken fat
to taste
Freshly ground black pepper

Preheat oven to 275°.

Cook bacon until crisp. Reserve fat.

Place 2 tablespoons of bacon fat in a frying pan. Sauté
chicken livers until they are pink inside.

Season chicken cutlet with 1 teaspoon salt, and sauté in
butter for 3 minutes on each side. Add wine and simmer for
5 minutes.

Put bacon, chicken livers, chicken, water chestnuts, and
eggs into a large wooden chopping bowl or food processor
and chop fine.

Add remaining seasoned salt, Boursin cheese, basil, chicken
fat, and pepper. Mix well. Place mixture in a small loaf pan.
Pack down well. Put a heavy weight on top to keep the pâté
from rising.

Bake for 2 hours. Open the oven door and cook for one
hour more. Remove from oven and allow to come to room
temperature. Refrigerate.

Makes 20 servings.

1.6 GRAMS PER SERVING

Mother's Chopped Liver

1 pound chicken livers
3 tablespoons chicken fat
½ medium Bermuda onion,
   cut into 4 pieces

2 hard-boiled eggs, quartered
2 teaspoons seasoned salt
Freshly cracked black pepper
   to taste

Sauté chicken livers in 2 tablespoons chicken fat for about 3 minutes on each side.

Remove to a wooden chopping bowl. Add onions and eggs. Chop well. Spoon in remaining chicken fat and sprinkle with seasoned salt and pepper. Blend well and refrigerate.

Makes 8 servings for appetizers.

Makes 16 servings for hors d'oeuvres.

2.2 GRAMS PER APPETIZER
1.1 GRAMS PER HORS D'OEUVRE

Avocado Cream Mold

1 package diet lime gelatin
¾ cup boiling water
1 cup sour cream
1 ripe avocado, peeled and
   mashed

1 tablespoon lemon juice
1 package sugar substitute
   (brown, if possible)
¼ teaspoon Worcestershire
   sauce

Dissolve gelatin in boiling water. Cool to room temperature. With a wooden spoon, stir in sour cream. Add avocado, lemon juice, sugar substitute, and Worcestershire sauce. Stir until mixture is smooth and creamy. Pour into a 4-cup mold and chill until firm.

Makes 4 servings.

6.2 GRAMS PER SERVING

Avocado Spread

½ avocado
2 tablespoons ground toasted
    sesame seeds

1 teaspoon lemon juice
½ teaspoon salt

Mash avocado, add ground seeds, lemon juice, and salt.
Blend well.
    Use to stuff celery.
    Makes 2 servings.

6.4 GRAMS PER SERVING

Guacamole

1 avocado, peeled and
    chopped
½ cup chopped onion
1 tomato, chopped
½ cucumber, peeled and
    chopped
½ teaspoon seasoned salt

1 teaspoon Salad Supreme
Freshly ground black pepper
1 tablespoon sour cream
1 tablespoon lecithin
    granules
1 tablespoon chopped
    parsley

Place avocado, onion, tomato, and cucumber in a bowl and
mix together. Season with salt, Salad Supreme and pepper.
Add sour cream, lecithin granules, and parsley. Refrigerate.
    Makes 2 cups.

TOTAL GRAMS 31.0
15.5 GRAMS PER CUP

Tuna Spread

1 3-ounce package cream cheese
3 tablespoons mayonnaise
1 tablespoon minced onion
1 small clove garlic, minced
½ teaspoon celery seed

1 teaspoon horseradish
½ teaspoon Worcestershire sauce
½ teaspoon seasoned salt
1 6½- or 7-ounce can tuna fish

Combine all ingredients except tuna fish in a small bowl. Blend well with a fork.
    Drain tuna fish, crumble and add to mayonnaise mixture. Blend well.
    Makes 1¼ cups.

TOTAL GRAMS 4.6

Clam Dip

2 8-ounce packages cream cheese, softened
1 teaspoon seasoned salt
2 teaspoons Worcestershire sauce

4½-ounce can minced clams, with juice
1 teaspoon onion flakes

Put all ingredients in a bowl and mix thoroughly.
    Refrigerate for 10 minutes.

TOTAL GRAMS 6.6

Holiday Stuffed Edam (Gouda) Cheese

1 whole 10-ounce Edam
    (Gouda) cheese
8 ounces cream cheese,
    softened

4-ounce combination of
    smoked oysters and/or
    clams, minced
4 thin strips pimiento
12 stuffed olives

Scoop out center of cheese and reserve. Leave ⅛- to ¼-inch shell with red covering peel on. Grate center of cheese finely.

In blender combine grated cheese, cream cheese, oysters, and clams. Blend thoroughly.

Loosely spoon into cheese shell. Use back of spoon to form slight peaks. Decorate with pimiento strips. Arrange olives on toothpicks around rim of cheese for garnish.

Makes 8 servings.

2.7 GRAMS PER SERVING

Dip It

1 pound creamed cottage
    cheese
2 tablespoons white horse-
    radish
1 teaspoon seasoned salt

1 teaspoon garlic powder
1 teaspoon dried tarragon
½ teaspoon cayenne pepper
½ teaspoon dry mustard
½ teaspoon celery seed

Combine all ingredients and refrigerate for at least 3 hours. Serve with raw vegetables cut into bite-sized pieces.

Makes 2 cups or 8 servings.

1.9 GRAMS PER SERVING (¼ cup)

Cheese Ball 1

3 ounces cream cheese
½ teaspoon garlic powder
3 tablespoons sunflower
    seeds

Brie cheese
2 slices boiled ham
Boursin cheese
½ cup chopped walnuts

Sprinkle cream cheese with garlic powder. Shape into a ball and roll in sunflower seeds. Discard the white skin of enough Brie to cover ball and wrap the ham around the Brie. Cover the ham with Boursin and roll the entire ball in chopped walnuts.

    Refrigerate for at least 2 hours.
    Makes 6 servings.

3.1 GRAMS PER SERVING

Cheese Ball 2

2 tablespoons Roquefort
    cheese
4 tablespoons cream cheese
2 tablespoons sesame seeds

Brie at room temperature
¼ cup pine nuts
Dash cayenne pepper
Freshly chopped parsley

Combine Roquefort cheese and cream cheese. Form into a ball. Roll in sesame seeds. Take the white skin off enough Brie to cover ball. Roll Brie-covered ball in pine nuts, sprinkle with cayenne, and then roll in parsley.

    Makes 6 servings.

TOTAL GRAMS 23.9
3.9 GRAMS PER SERVING

Clams Casino

2 dozen clams	1 large tomato, sliced
¼ cup white wine	4 strips bacon, fried and
2 tablespoons butter	crumbled
1 small onion, minced	Grated Parmesan cheese

Preheat broiler.

Steam clams in white wine until they open. Remove half of the clam shell, leaving clams intact.

Sauté onion in butter until golden. Spoon sautéed onion over clams. Add tomato and bacon. Sprinkle with Parmesan cheese.

Place under a hot broiler until the cheese is melted.

Makes 6 appetizer servings.

2.9 GRAMS PER SERVING

Marbleized Tea Eggs from China

6 eggs	2 tablespoons soy sauce
2 tablespoons salt	3 tablespoons black tea
1 tablespoon anise extract	

Cover eggs with cold water and bring to a boil. Simmer 10 minutes.

Remove eggs, cool, and crack the shells in several places, but do not peel.

Bring to a boil 4 cups of water. Add remaining ingredients and eggs. Simmer for 1 hour. Cool.

Place eggs still in the water in the refrigerator. Leave overnight.

To serve, shell eggs, cut in half or quarters, or leave them whole. They are very attractive on the hors d'oeuvres tray.

TOTAL GRAMS 2.3

Green Onion and Red Caviar Quiche

1 10-inch pie plate
Baked Pie Crust 1
    (optional, page 124)
2 tablespoons chicken fat
6 green onions, chopped
Seasoned salt and pepper to
    taste
1 whole egg

2 egg yolks
1 teaspoon Dijon mustard
½ teaspoon dry mustard
½ cup grated Swiss cheese
1½ cups heavy cream
2 ounces red caviar
2 tablespoons minced parsley

Preheat oven to 300°.

Melt chicken fat. Add green onions and sauté for 5 minutes. Season with salt and pepper.

Make a custard by mixing eggs, mustards, and Swiss cheese.

Scald the cream by bringing it just to the boiling point (do not boil).

Combine the green onion mixture with the custard and cream. Mix well and pour into pie plate. Bake for 45 minutes.

Remove from oven. Spread top with caviar. Sprinkle with parsley. Serve.

Makes 10 servings.

6.9 GRAMS PER SERVING WITH CRUST
2.7 GRAMS PER SERVING WITHOUT CRUST

Roquefort Quiche

3 ounces Roquefort cheese
6 ounces cream cheese or
    cottage cheese
2 tablespoons softened butter
3 tablespoons heavy cream
2 eggs

½ teaspoon minced fresh
    chives or ½ teaspoon
    minced scallion
Cayenne pepper to taste
Salt and white pepper to
    taste

Preheat oven to 375°.

Blend the cheeses, butter, and cream with a fork; then beat in the eggs.

Force the mixture through a sieve, to smooth. Season to taste and stir in the chives or scallion.

Pour into pie plate (or crust) and set in upper third of oven.

Bake for 25-30 minutes, or until top has puffed and browned.

Makes 6 servings.

1.3 GRAMS PER SERVING

Zucchini Parmesan Quiche

1 10-inch pie plate or Pie
    Crust 1, 2, or 3
    (optional, see Index)
2 tablespoons sweet butter
1 tablespoon olive oil
½ large zucchini, sliced thin
1 small tomato, chopped
¼ teaspoon garlic powder

Salt and pepper to taste
1 egg, plus 2 egg yolks
1 teaspoon Dijon mustard
½ teaspoon dry mustard
½ cup grated Parmesan
    cheese
½ cup heavy cream

Preheat oven to 300°.

Melt butter and add olive oil. Sauté zucchini until transparent. Add tomato, garlic powder, salt, and pepper. Cook for 3 minutes.

Beat the eggs, mustards, and Parmesan cheese until mixture is thickened.

Scald the cream by bringing it just to the boiling point. Do not boil. Add the cream, in droplets, to the egg mixture, beating constantly, Fold in the zucchini mixture, mix well, and pour into pie plate.

Bake for 45 minutes.

Makes 10 servings.

5.1 GRAMS PER SERVING WITH CRUST
1.4 GRAMS PER SERVING WITHOUT CRUST

Muenster Quiche

1 10-inch pie plate
3 tablespoons sweet butter
½ cup sliced mushrooms
1 cup fresh spinach leaves
Salt and pepper to taste
1 egg plus 2 egg yolks

1 teaspoon Dijon mustard
½ teaspoon dry mustard
¼ pound grated Muenster cheese
1½ cups heavy cream

Preheat oven to 300°.

Melt butter. Add mushrooms, spinach, salt, and pepper. Sauté until mushrooms are golden.

Beat the eggs, mustards, and Muenster cheese until mixture is thickened. Scald the cream by bringing it just to the boiling point. Do not boil. Add it to the egg mixture in droplets, beating constantly.

Fold in the spinach mixture, mix well, and pour into pie plate.

Bake for 45 minutes.
Makes 8 servings.

TOTAL GRAMS WITHOUT CRUST 23.4
2.9 GRAMS PER SERVING

The Cream of Clams

2 dozen clams
½ cup dry white wine
1 small onion, minced
2 tablespoons butter

½ cup heavy cream
2 tablespoons grated Parmesan cheese
½ teaspoon seasoned salt

Preheat oven to 350°.

Steam the clams in the wine. Remove clams from shells, reserving half of the shell. Chop the clams.

Sauté onion in butter until golden.

Combine the clams, onion, cream, Parmesan cheese, and salt. Blend well over a low flame. Return creamed mixture to shells and bake for 15 minutes.

Makes 6 appetizer servings.

1.5 GRAMS PER APPETIZER SERVING

Chicken Livers and Water Chestnuts

18 slices bacon (without nitrate if possible)	9 water chestnuts, sliced into 4 slices each
	9 chicken livers, quartered

Cut bacon in half. Place 1 piece each of water chestnut and chicken liver at end of bacon. Roll up. Freeze. When ready to serve, do not defrost. Broil for 3 minutes on each side or until bacon is of desired doneness.

Makes 36 hors d'oeuvres.

0.9 GRAM PER HORS D'OEUVRE

Stuffed Cucumber Sticks

2 large cucumbers	1 tablespoon minced pimiento
2 6-ounce packages frozen Alaska king crab, thawed and well drained	2 teaspoons lemon juice
½ cup mayonnaise	½ teaspoon seasoned salt
½ cup celery	Dash Tabasco sauce
	Lettuce leaves

Peel and halve cucumber lengthwise; spoon out the seeds and salt well.

In a small bowl mix together the remaining ingredients, except the lettuce.

Fill the cucumber halves with crab mixture and serve on lettuce leaves.

Makes 4 servings.

3.2 GRAMS PER SERVING

Little Meatballs for Soup or Appetizers

2 tablespoons butter
1 small onion, minced
1 medium stalk of celery, minced
1 clove garlic, minced
½ pound ground beef
½ cup Hi-Protein bread crumbs

1 egg
½ teaspoon thyme
1 teaspoon seasoned salt
¼ teaspoon pepper
1 tablespoon grated Parmesan cheese
¼ teaspoon curry powder (optional)

Heat butter in a small skillet. Sauté onion, celery, and garlic until golden brown.

Place beef in a bowl, add onion mixture and remaining ingredients. Mix lightly with a fork. Shape into 1-inch balls. Drop into boiling soup for 10 minutes.

Makes 8 meatballs.

FOR APPETIZERS: Prepare as in preceding recipe. Shape into 1-inch balls and sauté. Place a toothpick in each before serving.

3.7 TOTAL GRAMS PER MEATBALL

Crabmeat Cocktail

1 6½-ounce can crabmeat
3 tablespoons mayonnaise
2 tablespoons tomato sauce
1 tablespoon horseradish
2 drops Tabasco

2 tablespoons minced celery
2 tablespoons minced onion
2 tablespoons minced green
    pepper
Lettuce leaves

Combine all ingredients and blend well. Chill.
    Serve on lettuce leaves.
    Makes 2 servings.

3.9 GRAMS PER SERVING

Pink Seafood Cocktail

2 cups seafood: crab, shrimp,
    lobster, or salmon
1 cup mayonnaise
½ cup tomato sauce

2 tablespoons lemon juice
2 teaspoons celery seed
3 or 4 drops Tabasco
Dash salt

Remove any shell or skin from seafood. Remove vein from
back of shrimp.
    Combine the rest of the ingredients. Chill.
    Serve in cocktail glasses, or on lettuce leaves, with sauce
on top.
    Makes 6 servings.

2.8 GRAMS PER SERVING

Mushrooms Stuffed with Shrimp

1 pound cooked, shelled, and
    deveined shrimp
1 pound large mushrooms,
    stemmed
½ cup lemon juice
¼ cup wine vinegar

½ cup olive oil
1 teaspoon garlic salt
1 teaspoon oregano
1 8-ounce package cream
    cheese with chives,
    softened

Combine lemon juice, wine vinegar, olive oil, garlic salt, and oregano in a large bowl. Add shrimp and mushrooms and refrigerate marinade for 5 to 6 hours, stirring occasionally.

Stir cream cheese until smooth.

Drain shrimp and mushrooms. Fill each mushroom cap with about 1 tablespoon of cream cheese. Top with shrimp.

Makes about 20 mushrooms.

1.7 GRAMS PER MUSHROOM

Soups and Soup Stocks

Beef Soup Stock

2 pounds beef plate
1 tablespoon salt
3 quarts cold water
¼ teaspoon pepper
¼ cup diced onion
¼ cup diced carrot

¼ cup diced celery
¼ cup diced tomato
1 teaspoon chopped parsley
1 teaspoon chopped green
    pepper

Place meat and salt in cold water, and bring to a boil over low heat. Skim off the top. Cover and simmer for 2½ hours.

Add the vegetables, seasonings and pepper, and cook slowly for an additional 1½ hours.

Remove the meat and serve with horseradish or mustard sauce. Strain the stock and use as directed in recipes.

Makes 2 quarts.

0.7 GRAMS PER SERVING

Quick Court Bouillon

2 tablespoons butter
3 sprigs fresh parsley, or 1
    teaspoon dried parsley
    flakes
1 large onion, sliced
1 large carrot, sliced

3 stalks celery, sliced
2 quarts water
6 whole black peppercorns
2 whole cloves
1 bay leaf
2 tablespoons wine vinegar

Melt butter in deep saucepan over medium flame. Add vegetables and sauté 5 minutes. Add water and seasonings, cover tightly, and simmer for 30 minutes.

Strain and use as directed in recipes.

Makes 2 quarts.

2.1 GRAMS PER SERVING

Fish Stock with Spices

2 pounds fish trimmings	1 parsley sprig
2 quarts water	1 bay leaf
2 cloves	5 peppercorns
½ teaspoon mace	1 tablespoon salt
3 stalks celery, with tops	

Place all ingredients in deep saucepan. Cover tightly and bring to a boil. Lower flame and simmer gently for 45 minutes. Strain, cool, and store in refrigerator. Use as directed in recipes.

Makes 3 pints.

6 GRAMS PER SERVING

Plain Fish Stock

Just use trimmings, water, bay leaf, and salt. Place in covered saucepan and simmer for 30 minutes. Strain and store in refrigerator.

TRACE PER SERVING

Consommé

1 pound lean beef, cubed	½ cup sliced onion
1 pound veal bones	½ cup sliced carrots
1 pound marrow bones	½ cup sliced celery
1 pound beef bones	2 tablespoons oil
2 pounds chicken, cleaned and cut up	1 tablespoon salt
	¼ teaspoon pepper
6 quarts cold water	¼ teaspoon nutmeg

Heat skillet and brown beef on all sides. Place water in large pot and add bones, chicken, and browned beef. Bring to a boil quickly and skim off the top. Cover and simmer for several hours.

Fry the vegetables in oil for a few minutes and add to the soup with seasonings. Boil for another hour.

Strain, cool, and skim off the fat.

Chicken and beef may be used in separate dishes calling for boiled meat. Soup can be used as stock when called for in recipes or can be eaten with soup garnishes.

Makes 5 quarts.

1.2 GRAMS SERVING

Chicken Broth

1 4-pound stewing chicken	1 bay leaf
1 onion	Pinch of thyme
1 stalk celery	¼ teaspoon pepper
1 sprig parsley	⅛ teaspoon nutmeg
3 carrots	

Wash and clean the chicken. Place it in a large pot and cover with water. Bring to boil and add vegetables and seasonings. Simmer gently for 2 hours.

Cool, strain, and use as soup or broth.
Makes 1 quart.

VARIATION: Turkey soup may be made the same way by using a cut-up turkey carcass instead of stewing chicken. The larger the amount of turkey bones, the more flavorful the soup.

5.5 GRAMS PER SERVING

Egg Drop Soup

8 cups chicken broth
½ pound washed, trimmed, and chopped spinach
¼ cup finely sliced scallions

3 eggs
½ teaspoon garlic powder
¼ teaspoon seasoned salt

Bring chicken stock to a boil over moderate heat. Add spinach and boil mixture for 5 minutes. Stir in the scallions.

Combine the eggs with the garlic and salt; beat lightly to combine. Add mixture in a steady stream to soup. Stir the soup and let simmer for 2 minutes.
Makes 6 servings.

1.8 GRAMS PER SERVING

Garlic Soup

16 cloves garlic
2 quarts water
2 teaspoons salt
Pinch pepper
2 cloves
¼ teaspoon sage
¼ teaspoon thyme

½ bay leaf
4 parsley sprigs
7 tablespoons olive oil
3 egg yolks
1 cup grated Parmesan cheese

Drop garlic cloves in boiling water for 30 seconds. Drain, run cold water over them, and peel.

Place the garlic, water, salt, pepper, cloves, sage, thyme, bay leaf, parsley, and 3 tablespoons olive oil in a saucepan, and boil slowly for 30 minutes. Correct seasoning.

Beat the egg yolks in a soup tureen for a minute, until they are thick and sticky. Slowly pour in 4 tablespoons olive oil, drop by drop, beating constantly until the sauce has thickened.

Beat a ladleful of hot soup into the egg mixture by droplets. Gradually strain in the rest, beating, and pressing the juice out of the garlic. Sprinkle with Parmesan cheese and serve immediately.

Makes 8 servings.

2.6 GRAMS PER SERVING

Italian Clam Soup

4 dozen littleneck clams	1 tablespoon tomato paste
¼ cup olive oil	1½ cups warm water
1 clove garlic	½ teaspoon salt
3 chopped anchovy fillets	½ teaspoon freshly ground
1 tablespoon chopped parsley	black pepper
½ cup dry red wine	¼ teaspoon oregano

Wash the clams and scrub well with a vegetable brush.

Place the oil in a large saucepan, add the garlic, and brown. Discard the garlic. Add the anchovies, parsley, and wine to the oil and cook 5 minutes.

Add the tomato paste, water, salt, and pepper, and cook 3-4 minutes.

Add the clams, cover the pan, and cook until all the shells are open—a maximum of 5 minutes. Add the oregano and cook 2 minutes longer.

Pour into large, shallow soup dishes and serve immediately.
Makes 4 servings.

5.9 GRAMS PER SERVING

Cucumber Soup

2 cups chicken broth
½ cup dry white wine
¼ cup water
1 tablespoon lemon juice

¼ cup cream
1 cucumber, unpared, sliced
   very thin

Combine first 5 ingredients in a blender until smooth. Add sliced cucumber.
   Serve either heated or chilled.
   Makes 4 servings.

3.2 GRAMS PER SERVING

Cold Avocado Soup

1½ cups diced, peeled avocado
3 tablespoons lime juice
½ teaspoon salt
Dash pepper

Dash nutmeg
2 12½-ounce cans chicken
   broth
¼ cup heavy cream,
   whipped

Place avocado, lime juice, salt, pepper, and nutmeg in a blender. Add 1 can chicken broth. Blend 30 seconds at high speed. Pour into bowl.
   Stir in remaining 1 can broth and chill until ice-cold.
   Serve garnished with a spoonful of whipped cream and a sprinkling of nutmeg.
   Makes 6 servings.

5.1 GRAMS PER SERVING

Cream of Sorrel Soup

½ pound sorrel, finely
   chopped
1 teaspoon butter

5 cups chicken broth
4 egg yolks
2 cups light cream

Sauté the sorrel in butter until wilted. Set aside.

Bring the broth to a boil and remove from heat. Lightly beat together the egg yolks and cream, and add to broth by droplets, stirring vigorously with a whisk.

Return to low heat, stirring constantly, until slightly thickened. Do not boil.

Remove from heat, add the sorrel, and refrigerate. Stir often and serve cold.

Makes 8 servings.

5.5 GRAMS PER SERVING

New England Fish Chowder

2 pounds cod fillets
4 slices bacon, diced
2 small onions, diced
2 tablespoons chopped
   parsley

2 cups hot water
1 bay leaf
1 teaspoon salt
⅛ teaspoon pepper
1 quart heavy cream

Cut fish fillets into 1-inch cubes. Place bacon in deep saucepan over low heat and sauté until golden brown. Add onions and sauté until transparent. Add parsely and cook 1 minute more.

Add water, bay leaf, salt, and pepper. Cover and cook for a few minutes to combine flavors. Add fish, and simmer for 10 minutes. Add cream and heat to the boiling point. Do not boil. Serve immediately.

Makes 8 servings.

4.0 GRAMS PER SERVING

New England Clam Chowder

Wash 3 dozen clams thoroughly. Steam in covered pot in 4-6 inches of boiling water until shells open (no longer than 5 minutes). Strain clam broth and use as part of water in recipe. Chop clams coarsely and substitute for fish fillets.

Makes 6-8 servings.

4.3 GRAMS PER SERVING

Egg Dishes

Basic Omelet

2 tablespoons butter
4 eggs
1 tablespoon heavy cream

½ teaspoon seasoned salt
Freshly cracked black pepper

Melt butter in omelet pan and tilt pan to cover well.

Beat eggs with cream, salt, and pepper. Pour into pan and tilt pan to spread to edges of pan.

Cook over a low flame until eggs begin to set. Loosen eggs from sides of pan with a spatula. Tilt pan again to allow uncooked egg to go to the sides. Carefully fold the outer edges of the omelet into the middle to resemble a flat cone.

Slide omelet out of pan and serve.

Makes 2 servings.

0.7 GRAM PER SERVING

Blintz Omelet

8 eggs
½ cup creamed cottage
    cheese
½ cup cream cheese,
    softened
Pinch salt
2 packets sugar substitute

1 teaspoon vanilla
½ teaspoon cinnamon
¼ cup heavy cream
3 tablespoons butter
2 tablespoons sour cream
    (optional)

Combine all ingredients except butter and sour cream in a bowl and beat until smooth.

Melt butter in a large omelet pan. Pour egg mixture into omelet pan and tilt the pan to spread mixture to edges. Cook over a low heat until eggs begin to set. Loosen eggs from sides of pan with a spatula. Tilt pan again to allow uncooked egg mixture to spread to the sides. When center is firm, carefully fold two of the outer edges of the omelet into the center to resemble a flat cone.

Slide out of pan and serve plain or with sour cream on the side.

Makes 4 servings.

4.2 GRAMS PER SERVING

Creamy Peach Omelet

1 8-ounce package cream cheese, softened	¼ cup heavy cream
8 eggs	1 packet sugar substitute
Pinch salt	2 tablespoons butter
	⅓ cup diet peach jam

Combine all ingredients except butter and jam in a bowl and beat until smooth.

Melt butter in a large omelet pan. Pour egg mixture into omelet pan and tilt the pan to spread mixture to edges. Cook over a low heat until eggs begin to set. Loosen eggs from sides of pan with a spatula. Tilt pan again to allow uncooked egg mixture to spread to the sides. When center is firm, spoon jam onto the center of the omelet. Carefully fold two of the outer edges of the omelet into the center to resemble a flat cone.

Slide out of pan and serve.

Makes 4 servings.

5.1 GRAMS PER SERVING

Alfalfa and Cheddar Cheese Omelet

3 tablespoons alfalfa sprouts   4 eggs
4 tablespoons grated   1 tablespoon heavy cream
   Cheddar cheese   1 teaspoon seasoned salt
2 tablespoons butter   Freshly cracked black pepper

Combine alfalfa sprouts and Cheddar cheese. Melt butter in
an omelet pan. Beat eggs with cream, salt, and pepper. Fold
alfalfa mixture into eggs. Pour into omelet pan and tilt to
spread eggs to edges of pan. Cook over a low flame until eggs
begin to set. Loosen eggs from sides of pan with a spatula.
Tilt pan again to allow uncooked egg mixture to spread to
the edges.

Carefully fold the outer edges of the omelet into the center
to resemble a flat cone. Slide omelet out of pan and serve.
Makes 2 servings.

This may be served as it is, or with a ham and mushroom
filling.

0.8 GRAM PER SERVING

Boursin and Lecithin Omelet

3 tablespoons Boursin cheese   4 eggs
1 tablespoon lecithin gran-   1 tablespoon heavy cream
   ules   1 teaspoon seasoned salt
2 tablespoons butter   Freshly cracked black pepper

Cream Boursin and lecithin together with the back of a
spoon.

Melt butter in omelet pan. Beat eggs with cream, salt, and
pepper. Break Boursin up and beat it into the eggs. Pour mixture into an omelet pan and tilt the pan to spread the mixture
to the edges of the pan.

Cook over a low flame until eggs begin to set. Loosen eggs from sides of pan with spatula. Tilt pan to allow uncooked egg mixture to spread to the sides.

Carefully fold the outer edges of the omelet into the center to resemble a flat cone. Slide omelet out of pan and serve.

Makes 2 servings.

This may be served with a caviar and watercress filling.

1.2 GRAMS PER SERVING

Reuben Omelet

2 tablespoons butter	1 tablespoon brown mustard
4 eggs	⅛ pound corned beef
1 tablespoon heavy cream	4 slices Swiss cheese
Seasoned salt	1 tablespoon hot sauerkraut
Freshly cracked black pepper	

Melt butter in an omelet pan. Beat eggs with cream, salt, and pepper. Pour into omelet pan and tilt to spread eggs to edges of pan. Cook over a low flame until eggs begin to set. Tilt pan again to allow uncooked egg to spread to edges. Spread mustard down center of omelet.

Break up beef and Swiss cheese into bite-sized pieces and add to the pan.

Carefully fold the outer edges of the omelet into the center to resemble a flat cone. Slide omelet out of pan and serve topped with hot sauerkraut.

Makes 2 servings.

3.9 GRAMS PER SERVING

French Toast

1 tablespoon butter	Dash salt
1 egg, slightly beaten	6 slices Hi-Protein Soya
¼ cup cream	bread
½ teaspoon vanilla extract	Cinnamon

Heat butter in a heavy skillet.

Place the egg, cream, vanilla, salt, and ¼ cup water in a small bowl. Blend with a fork.

Dip bread into egg mixture and sauté in butter on both sides to a golden brown. Sprinkle each slice with cinnamon.

Makes 6 servings.

3.6 GRAMS PER SERVING

Fish Soufflé

2 tablespoons butter	1 cup flaked, cooked, or
3 tablespoons soya flour	canned fish
1 teaspoon salt	¼ teaspoon onion juice
1 cup heavy cream, heated	3 eggs, separated
	1⅓ tablespoons lemon juice

Preheat oven to 350°.

Melt the butter and stir in the flour and salt. Whisk vigorously for 1 full minute to avoid floury taste. Add the heated cream and cook over low heat, whisking, until thickened. Remove from heat and cool. Add the fish and onion juice, beat the egg yolks, and blend them into the mixture. Fold in stiffly beaten egg whites and lemon juice. Pour into greased soufflé dish or straight-sided casserole. Set in a pan of hot water, and bake about 35 minutes until firm. Serve immediately.

Makes 6 servings.

5.2 GRAMS PER SERVING

Spicy Cauliflower Soufflé

5 eggs, separated
1 cup grated Cheddar cheese
½ cup heavy cream
10-ounce package frozen
cauliflower, slightly
thawed (or fresh,
steamed 3 minutes),
chopped
¼ teaspoon onion salt
¼ teaspoon nutmeg
Dash cayenne pepper

Preheat oven to 350°.

Place all ingredients except egg whites in blender or food processor. Puree until smooth.

Beat egg whites until stiff peaks form. Fold into cauliflower mixture. Pour into greased soufflé dish.

Bake for 1 hour and serve immediately

Makes 4 servings.

5.6 GRAMS PER SERVING

Vegetable Soufflé

½ tablespoon finely chopped
onion
½ tablespoon finely chopped
green pepper
1 tablespoon finely chopped
celery
2 tablespoons melted butter
1 tablespoon arrowroot flour
½ cup heavy cream
½ teaspoon salt
Pinch white pepper
1 teaspoon parsley
1 teaspoon savory
¼ teaspoon sweet basil
¾ cup diced cooked vege-
tables (broccoli, cauli-
flower, cabbage, egg-
plant, green beans,
tomatoes)
3 eggs, separated

Preheat oven to 325°.

Lightly brown the onion, green pepper, and celery in butter. Blend in flour and cream. Cook over low heat, stirring constantly, until thickened. Season with herbs and spices and stir in vegetables. Add hot mixture gradually, in droplets, to beaten egg yolks, whisking constantly. Beat egg whites until stiff peaks form. Fold into vegetable mixture.

Pour into greased baking dish and bake about 1 hour, or until set.

Makes 4 servings.

4.3 GRAMS PER SERVING

CHEESE VEGETABLE SOUFFLÉ

Add 1 cup grated hard cheese and ¼ cup more cream to flour mixture before it thickens. Proceed with original recipe.

6.4 GRAMS PER SERVING

Winter Squash Soufflé

1 winter squash
2 packets sugar substitute
1 teaspoon cinnamon
½ cup butter
1 teaspoon salt
4 egg yolks
2 egg whites

Preheat oven to 350°.

Peel squash and dice. Place in water to cover and cover pot. Cook 20 minutes or until soft. Drain.

Add sugar substitute, cinnamon, butter, and salt. Mash with fork or puree with food mill or food processor.

Add egg yolks and mix well. Beat whites into stiff peaks. Fold gently into squash mixture. Pour into a greased soufflé dish with collar. Bake for 35 minutes.

Makes 6 servings.

3.0 GRAMS PER SERVING

Main Dishes

Baked Fish with Sour Cream

2 pounds fish fillets
1½ teaspoons seasoned salt
¼ teaspoon pepper
1 cup sour cream

3 tablespoons prepared
    horseradish
2 tablespoons grated lemon
    peel
1 teaspoon celery seed

Preheat oven to 325°.

Wash fillets, sprinkle with salt and pepper. Place fillets in an oiled baking dish.

Combine remaining ingredients and mix well. Pour over fillets.

Cover baking dish, or use aluminum foil and seal edges. Bake for 30 minutes.

Makes 6 servings.

4.9 GRAMS PER SERVING

Salmon Oregano

4 salmon steaks or salmon
    fillets
Salt and pepper to taste
4 tablespoons olive oil

1 large onion, minced
1 8-ounce can tomato sauce
Dash oregano

Wash salmon, sprinkle with salt and pepper.

Heat 2 tablespoons oil in a skillet. Sauté salmon until golden brown on each side, and remove to a warm dish.

71

In a skillet, heat the remainder of the oil and sauté onion until light brown. Add tomato sauce and oregano.

Simmer for 15 minutes.

Pour over salmon and serve.

Makes 4 servings.

4.4 GRAMS PER SERVING

Cheese Broiled Fish

1 pound fish fillets
1 teaspoon seasoned salt
¼ teaspoon pepper
4 tablespoons butter

1 recipe Cream Sauce
** (page 104)**
½ cup shredded Cheddar
** cheese**

Preheat broiler.

Wash fillets, rub with salt and pepper.

Oil a baking dish.

Place fillets in a single layer in the dish, dot with butter. Broil 5 minutes.

Pour Cream Sauce over fillets. Sprinkle cheese on top. Broil again until lightly brown.

Makes 2 servings.

4.1 GRAMS PER SERVING

Fish au Gratin

2 pounds flounder, sole, cod,
** haddock, or pike fillets**
1 teaspoon seasoned salt
¼ teaspoon paprika
3 tablespoons lemon juice

2 tablespoons butter
Cream Sauce (page 104)
½ cup grated cheese
Dash paprika

Place the fish in an oiled baking dish, sprinkle with salt, paprika, lemon juice, and butter. Cover, or use aluminum foil and seal the edges.

Bake about 25 minutes until fish flakes easily.

When fish is cooked, drain off any excess liquid. Pour Cream Sauce over the fish and sprinkle with cheese and paprika.

Makes 4 servings.

2.6 GRAMS PER SERVING

Fish Fillets with Scallop Sauce

9 tablespoons butter
½ pound scallops
1 pound fish fillets
Salt and pepper

1 cup sliced mushrooms
⅔ cup white wine
½ cup heavy cream

Heat 2 tablespoons of butter, and sauté scallops until light brown. Set aside.

Wash fish fillets and sprinkle with salt and pepper. Sauté in 4 tablespoons of butter until golden brown on each side. Turn with a spatula, being careful not to break the fillets.

Sauté mushrooms in 3 tablespoons of butter until slightly softened. Remove mushrooms and keep covered in warm dish. Add the wine and cook until sauce is reduced by half.

Add cream, scallops, and mushrooms. Stir and heat thoroughly, without bringing to a boil. Pour over fish and serve.

Makes 4 servings.

1.9 GRAMS PER SERVING

Peppered Fish

1 canned green chili pepper,
  or 1 mild cherry pepper
2 cloves garlic, minced
2 tablespoons lemon juice
3 tablespoons softened butter

1 tablespoon parsley
1 teaspoon seasoned salt
½ teaspoon black pepper
1 pound sole or flounder fillets

Preheat broiler.
   Clean the seeds from the pepper and mince.
   Combine with next 6 ingredients. Blend well.
   Spread mixture on both sides of fish. Marinate for 20 minutes. Broil for 10 minutes until flaky.
   Makes 4 servings.

2.0 GRAMS PER SERVING

Sicilian Fish

2 pounds sole, flounder,
  snapper, or bass fillets
½ teaspoon seasoned salt
½ teaspoon garlic salt
⅛ teaspoon pepper

1 cup grated Parmesan
  cheese
1 teaspoon basil
¼ cup butter

Preheat oven to 325°.
   Wash fish. Combine seasoned salt, garlic salt, and pepper. Rub into fish.
   Combine Parmesan cheese and basil. Coat fish with this mixture.
   Place fish in an oiled baking dish. Dot with butter. Bake about 25 minutes until fish flakes easily.
   Makes 4 servings.

1.2 GRAMS PER SERVING

Quick Poached Fish Fillets

2 pounds fish fillets
Boiling water to cover fish
1 small onion, chopped
½ cup white wine
1 teaspoon celery seed

2 bay leaves
2 tablespoons parsley
1 teaspoon seasoned salt
5 peppercorns

Wash fillets, place in a large skillet, cover with boiling water, and add remaining ingredients.

Cover and simmer 9 minutes, until fish flakes easily. Carefully remove fillets with a slotted spatula and arrange on a platter.

Serve with Parsley Butter (page 113) or Horseradish Sauce (page 106).

Makes 6 servings.

1.8 GRAMS PER SERVING

Scallops Sautéed

1 pound sea scallops
½ cup Hi-Protein bread
    crumbs
1 teaspoon seasoned salt
¼ teaspoon pepper

6 tablespoons butter
3 tablespoons lemon juice
1 tablespoon chopped parsley
1 tablespoon grated Parmesan cheese (optional)

Wash scallops.

Combine bread crumbs, salt, and pepper.

Heat butter in a pan. Sauté scallops until golden on all sides. Remove from pan with slotted spoon.

Add lemon juice and parsley to drippings in pan. Stir well and pour over scallops. Sprinkle with Parmesan cheese, if desired.

This can also be served on couscous or kasha.
Makes 2 servings.

8.8 GRAMS PER SERVING

Scallops with Green Sauce

2 pounds scallops	2 tablespoons butter
1 tablespoon seasoned salt	4 tablespoons dry white wine
4 tablespoons grated Parmesan cheese	1 recipe Green Sauce (page 104)

Wash and dry scallops. Sprinkle with salt and cheese. Sauté in butter for 3 minutes on each side. Lower heat, add wine, and simmer for 5 minutes. Add Green Sauce and continue to simmer for 2 more minutes.
Makes 4 servings.

2.8 GRAMS PER SERVING

Shrimp and Scallops Mark

½ pound medium shrimp	¼ cup heavy cream
Dash seasoned salt	2 tablespoons sweet butter
Dash garlic powder	3 strips bacon, quartered
1 egg, beaten	¼ cup dry white wine
¼ cup grated Parmesan cheese	¼ cup heavy cream
½ pound sea scallops	Tarragon

Sprinkle shrimp with salt and garlic powder. Dip shrimp in egg and then Parmesan cheese.

Sprinkle scallops with salt and garlic powder, dip into heavy cream and then into Parmesan cheese.

Melt butter in pan. Add bacon, scallops, and shrimp.

Brown on both sides; add wine and simmer for 10 minutes. Add cream and simmer gently for 10 minutes longer. Garnish with tarragon.

Makes 2 servings.

4.7 GRAMS PER SERVING

Mrs. Landau's Shrimp Sauté

4 tablespoons olive oil
1 pound raw shrimp, shelled
    and deveined
4 scallions, chopped
1 clove garlic, minced
Juice of 1 lemon

1 tablespoon chopped parsley
2 tablespoons blanched
    almonds
Seasoned salt and pepper to
    taste

Heat oil in skillet. Add shrimp, scallions, garlic, and lemon juice. Sauté until shrimp turn pink. Add parsley, almonds, salt, and pepper. Cook 1 minute longer.

Makes 3 servings.

3.5 GRAMS PER SERVING

Shrimp Marinara

2 pounds raw shrimp
2 tablespoons olive oil
½ cup minced onion
2 cloves garlic, minced
8 ounces tomato sauce

½ cup clam broth
1 teaspoon basil
¼ teaspoon oregano
2 teaspoons salt
Pepper to taste

Shell the shrimp and remove the vein down the back.

Heat oil in skillet. Sauté onion until golden, add garlic, and sauté 1 minute.

Add shrimp, sauté for 3 minutes.

Add tomato sauce, clam broth, basil, oregano, salt, and pepper.

Bring to a boil and simmer for 3 minutes.

Makes 4 servings.

6.9 GRAMS PER SERVING

Broiled Scampi

1 pound medium shrimp	**1 teaspoon garlic powder**
Juice of 1 lemon	**7 slices bacon**
¼ cup grated Parmesan cheese	

Preheat broiler.

Remove shells from shrimp and devein them. Squeeze the lemon juice on shrimp and allow to sit for 20 minutes.

Mix Parmesan cheese and garlic powder together. Dip shrimp in the mixture.

Place on a broiler pan and put ½ slice of bacon on each shrimp. Broil until shrimp turn bright pink.

Makes 3 servings.

1.8 GRAMS PER SERVING

Tony's Cream of Chicken

3 pounds chicken breasts, boned and skinned	**½ cup heavy cream**
Seasoned salt and pepper to taste	**¼ teaspoon nutmeg**
12 tablespoons butter	**½ cup grated Parmesan cheese**
3 egg yolks	**½ cup grated Swiss or Gruyère cheese**
½ cup water	**Dash paprika**

Preheat oven to 350°.

Sprinkle chicken with salt and pepper. Heat 4 tablespoons butter in a pan and brown chicken on all sides.

Place in a double boiler, over hot, not boiling water. Add the remaining butter and the egg yolks, one at a time. Beat constantly with rotary or electric beater. Add water, cream, and nutmeg. Beat until sauce thickens, about 6 minutes. Do not boil. Stir in Parmesan cheese, reserving 2 tablespoons to sprinkle on top. Add Swiss or Gruyère cheese.

Oil a baking dish and arrange the chicken in the bottom.

Spoon sauce over top of chicken. Sprinkle with remaining Parmesan cheese and paprika. Bake 30 minutes, or until golden brown.

Makes 4 servings.

2.2 GRAMS PER SERVING

Chicken India

4 chicken breasts, skinned	½ teaspoon seasoned salt
2 cloves garlic, crushed	¼ teaspoon black pepper
½ teaspoon grated fresh ginger or ¼ teaspoon ground ginger	1 egg, beaten
	¾ cup Hi-Protein bread crumbs
¼ teaspoon turmeric	3 tablespoons oil
2 tablespoons lemon juice	

Cut each chicken breast in half lengthwise and flatten.

Combine garlic, ginger, turmeric, lemon juice, salt, and pepper in a deep dish.

Rub the mixture into chicken breasts and chill for 3 hours.

Dip chicken breasts in egg, and roll in bread crumbs.

Heat oil in skillet and fry chicken about 10 minutes, or until crisp and golden. Drain on paper towels.

Makes 4 servings.

4.2 GRAMS PER SERVING

Chicken and Peaches

1 roasting chicken, 4 pounds	1 teaspoon ginger
1 cup sliced and peeled peaches	1 teaspoon seasoned salt
	½ teaspoon pepper
2 cups chicken broth	Juice of 2 limes
1 onion, peeled	4 ounces sugarless peach jam
4 cloves	
4 tablespoons butter	2 ounces Kirsch

Preheat oven to 375°.

Place peaches into a saucepan with chicken broth. Simmer for 5 minutes.

Wash and dry chicken thoroughly inside and out. Press cloves into onion and place into chicken cavity. Truss chicken.

Melt butter. Sprinkle ginger over chicken and rub in. Season with salt and pepper. Coat with melted butter. Roast, allowing 18 minutes per pound.

Remove chicken and carve into serving pieces. Keep warm. Pour off fat from roasting pan and scrape to loosen all particles. Add lime juice and peach jam. Simmer on top of stove until jam melts. Add Kirsch. Pour sauce over chicken and serve.

Makes 6 servings.

5.7 GRAMS PER SERVING

Chicken Breasts Divan

4 chicken breasts, skinned, boned and flattened	3 tablespoons butter
½ head broccoli flowerets	1 medium onion, finely chopped
Salt and pepper	1 cup grated Cheddar cheese
1 teaspoon garlic powder	½ pint sour cream
3 tablespoons minced parsley	

Preheat oven to 350°.

Boil broccoli for 5 minutes. Drain well.

Sprinkle chicken breasts with salt, pepper, garlic powder, and parsley.

Heat butter in a pan and sauté chicken breasts and onion until the onion is golden. Remove from pan and cut breasts into cubes.

Combine broccoli, chicken breasts, and Cheddar cheese. Blend well.

Put into a buttered casserole dish. Top with sour cream. Bake for ½ hour.

Makes 4 servings.

6.0 GRAMS PER SERVING

Chicken Breasts in Mushrooms and Cream

¼ pound sliced mushrooms	¼ cup beef bouillon
5 tablespoons butter	¼ cup dry Vermouth
4 chicken breasts, boned and skinned	1 cup heavy cream
2 tablespoons lemon juice	Salt and pepper to taste

Preheat oven to 400°.

Sauté mushrooms in butter until softened. Remove to a warm cup and cover tightly.

Rub chicken breasts with lemon juice, then roll in bubbling butter 1 minute on each side.

Transfer butter and chicken to heavy, ovenproof pot, cover top layer with a buttered circle of waxed paper, cover pot with a tight lid, and bake 5 minutes.

Remove chicken to warm platter and cover with mushrooms.

Add bouillon and wine to butter in pot and boil down rapidly, while whisking. Add cream and boil down 1 minute more. Remove from stove and season with lemon juice, salt, and pepper.

Pour sauce over chicken and mushrooms. Serve immediately.

Makes 4 servings.

5.0 GRAMS PER SERVING

Chicken Rolatini

4 chicken breasts, cut in half
    and boned
½ teaspoon seasoned salt
16 slices prosciutto or ham
1 8-ounce package Mozza-
    rella cheese
½ cup Hi-Protein bread
    crumbs
¼ teaspoon nutmeg
1 egg, slightly beaten with
    1 tablespoon cream
4 tablespoons butter
⅓ cup white wine
4 tablespoons grated Parme-
    san cheese

Pound chicken with mallet to break down membranes.

Sprinkle salt on chicken.

Place 2 slices of prosciutto and 1 tablespoon Mozzarella cheese inside each half chicken breast. Combine bread crumbs and nutmeg. Dip breast in egg, then in crumbs. Roll up the breast. Secure with a toothpick.

Heat butter in a large skillet until it foams. Add chicken rolls, and sauté until golden brown.

Pour wine over chicken rolls.

Sprinkle with Parmesan cheese. Cover and simmer for 20 minutes.

Makes 4 servings.

4.4 GRAMS PER SERVING

Swiss Chicken

1 chicken, cut into 8 pieces	½ cup white wine
Seasoned salt to taste	½ pound mushrooms,
Freshly cracked white pepper	sliced and sautéed in
to taste	butter
3 tablespoons butter	8 slices Swiss cheese

Preheat broiler.

Wash and dry the chicken. Sprinkle with salt and pepper.

Melt butter in skillet. Add chicken pieces and brown well on all sides. Pour wine over chicken. Cover pan and allow to simmer for ½ hour.

Just before serving, remove chicken to a baking dish. Cover chicken with sautéed mushrooms and top with cheese slices. Place under broiler until the cheese is brown and bubbly.

Makes 4 servings.

4.5 GRAMS PER SERVING

Chicken and Egg Loaf

¼ pound chicken livers	1 hard-boiled egg, chopped
2 tablespoons chicken fat	2 teaspoons lemon juice
¼ cup peanut oil	1 teaspoon Tabasco
6 eggs, lightly beaten	¼ teaspoon rosemary
1½ cups cooked and minced	¼ teaspoon basil
chicken	½ teaspoon seasoned salt
12 green olives, pitted and	½ teaspoon black pepper
finely chopped	

Preheat oven to 325°.

Sauté chicken livers in chicken fat for 6 minutes. Puree in blender with oil.

Place the mixture in a large bowl and stir in remaining ingredients.

Grease a loaf pan. Pour the mixture into the pan and bake for 45 minutes. Cut into slices and serve warm.

Makes 6 servings.

1.0 GRAM PER SERVING

Zucchini and Chicken

4 medium zucchini	**3 tablespoons sweet butter**
4 chicken breasts, boned and flattened	**¼ cup dry white wine**
	½ pint heavy cream
Salt and pepper to taste	**4 tablespoons grated Cheddar cheese**
Garlic powder	
½ cup grated Parmesan cheese	

Preheat oven to 400.°

Parboil zucchini for 5 minutes. Cut in half lengthwise and scoop out pulp.

Sprinkle chicken breasts with salt, pepper, garlic powder, and Parmesan cheese. Sauté the chicken breasts and zucchini pulp in butter until breasts are brown. Add wine and simmer 5 minutes. Remove from heat and chop in a wooden bowl. Add cream and return mixture to zucchini shells. Top with Cheddar cheese. Bake for ½ hour.

Makes 4 servings.

6.4 GRAMS PER SERVING

Beef Stroganoff

2 pounds sirloin or tender-
    loin steak, or rib steaks,
    cut in finger-size strips
6 tablespoons butter
1 large onion, sliced
½ pound mushrooms

½ cup beef broth
4 tablespoons tomato sauce
1 tablespoon dry sherry
1½ teaspoons seasoned salt
¼ teaspoon pepper
½ cup sour cream

Heat 3 tablespoons of butter and brown steak lightly. (Do not cook through.) Pour the drippings and meat into a bowl, and set aside.

In the same skillet, heat the remaining 3 tablespoons of butter, add the onion, and sauté for 3 minutes. Add mushrooms, and sauté until tender. Add beef broth, tomato sauce, sherry, salt, and pepper. Mix well. Place meat and drippings back in skillet with onion mixture. Cover, and simmer on very low heat for 15 minutes.

Add sour cream to sauce and blend well. Heat for 2 minutes more, do not boil.

Makes 6 servings.

3.6 GRAMS PER SERVING

English Hamburgers

1 pound chopped meat
4 tablespoons butter
½ cup chopped onion

½ teaspoon seasoned salt
½ teaspoon pepper
½ teaspoon dried sage

Melt 2 tablespoons butter in a skillet. Sauté onions until golden. Remove and set aside.

In same skillet, melt remaining 2 tablespoons butter. Add chopped meat, salt, pepper, and sage to the onions. Shape into patties.

Sauté hamburgers for 5 minutes on each side.
Makes 2 servings.

4.4 GRAMS PER SERVING

Greek Hamburgers

1 pound chopped meat
2 tablespoons butter
¼ cup crumbled feta cheese

¼ cup finely chopped black olives
½ teaspoon seasoned salt
½ teaspoon pepper

Melt the butter in a heavy pan.
   Mix the remaining ingredients and shape into patties.
   Sauté hamburgers for 5 minutes on each side.
   Makes 2 servings.

3.7 GRAMS PER SERVING

Indian Hamburgers

1 pound chopped meat
2 tablespoons butter
1 tablespoon finely chopped walnuts

2 teaspoons curry powder
½ teaspoon seasoned salt

Melt butter in a skillet.
   Mix the remainder of the ingredients and shape into patties.
   Sauté hamburgers for 5 minutes on each side.
   Makes 2 servings.

2.7 GRAMS PER SERVING

Italían Hamburgers

1 pound chopped meat	½ teaspoon seasoned salt
½ pound spinach, washed and drained	½ teaspoon pepper
2 tablespoons butter	1 tablespoon grated Parmesan cheese

Plunge spinach into boiling water and cook for 3 minutes. Drain and chop finely.

Melt butter in a skillet.

Mix the remainder of the ingredients with spinach and shape into patties.

Sauté hamburgers for 5 minutes on each side.

Makes 2 servings.

5.6 GRAMS PER SERVING

Spanish Hamburgers

1 pound chopped meat	½ teaspoon cumin
2 tablespoons butter	½ teaspoon chili powder
6 drops Tabasco Sauce	¼ teaspoon garlic powder

Melt butter in a skillet.

Mix the remainder of the ingredients and shape into patties.

Sauté hamburgers for 5 minutes on each side.

Makes 2 servings.

0.4 GRAM PER SERVING

U.S. Hamburgers

1 pound chopped meat	2 tablespoons butter
6 strips lean bacon	½ teaspoon seasoned salt
1 ripe tomato, finely chopped	½ teaspoon pepper

Fry bacon until crisp. Remove from pan, and spread over paper towels to drain and crisp. Crumble the bacon into a large bowl.

Sauté tomato in bacon grease until tender. Add it to the bacon.

Clean skillet and melt butter.

Combine chopped meat, salt, and pepper with bacon and tomato. Shape into patties.

Sauté hamburgers for 5 minutes on each side.
Makes 2 servings.

3.1 GRAMS PER SERVING

Meat Loaf Supreme

2 pounds freshly ground beef	Seasoned salt to taste
1 medium onion, sliced	3 hard-boiled eggs, sliced
2 tablespoons butter	1 small tomato, thinly sliced
¼ cup grated Cheddar cheese	1 egg, beaten

Preheat oven to 350°.

Sauté onion in butter until golden.

Mix onion, cheese, and salt with meat. Divide meat into two equal portions.

Place half of the meat in the bottom of an 8 × 8″ glass baking dish, pressing to cover the entire surface. Spread slices of egg and tomato on top. Cover with remaining meat. Make sure to press the meat together at the edges. Brush top with beaten egg.

Bake for 1 hour.

Makes 6 servings.

1.8 GRAMS PER SERVING

London Broil

1½ pounds London broil, cut ½-inch thick	2 tablespoons grated Parmesan cheese
1 teaspoon garlic powder	1 cup red wine
1½ teaspoons dry mustard	½ tablespoon black pepper

Preheat broiler.

Mix all ingredients and marinate for 2 hours.

Broil for 10 minutes on one side, 5, 7, or 9 minutes on the other side, depending on desired doneness.

Slice with the grain.

Makes 4–6 servings.

3.3 GRAMS PER SERVING

Steak au Poivre

4 shell steaks, pounded to ⅛-inch thickness	4 ounces cognac, warmed
Freshly ground black pepper	6 ounces heavy cream
6 tablespoons butter	2 teaspoons bottled steak sauce
2 teaspoons rosemary	2 teaspoons Dijon mustard
2 teaspoons sage	

Cover surface of steak on both sides with ground pepper. Press the pepper into the steak.

Melt butter and add rosemary and sage.

Add the steaks and brown quickly on both sides. Ignite warm cognac and pour over the steaks. When the fire goes out, remove steaks from the pan and keep warm.

Add the cream, steak sauce, and mustard to the pan juices. Stir well and simmer for 3 minutes. Pour over the steak and serve.

Makes 4 servings.

4.6 GRAMS PER SERVING

Greek Shish Kabob

2 cups safflower oil
1 cup lemon juice
2 tablespoons oregano
1 tablespoon garlic
4 bay leaves

1 teaspoon salt
1 teaspoon pepper
4–5-pound leg of lamb, cut into chunks
2 tomatoes, quartered

Preheat broiler.

In a large bowl place oil, lemon juice, oregano, garlic, bay leaves, salt, and pepper. Mix well. Add chunks of lamb and marinate for at least 2 hours, turning frequently. The longer the lamb marinates the better.

Remove lamb and place on skewers with quartered tomatoes. Place under broiler, basting with marinade and turning at frequent intervals, 20 minutes for medium and 30 minutes for well done.

Makes 6 servings.

5.3 GRAMS PER SERVING

Moussaka

1 medium eggplant
1½ pounds ground lamb or chuck
8 tablespoons sweet butter
3 egg yolks
1¼ cups water
¼ cup cream
½ cup grated Parmesan cheese
6 tablespoons olive oil

1 large onion, chopped
1 large green pepper, chopped
2 cloves garlic, minced
1 8-ounce can tomato sauce
1½ teaspoons cumin
¼ teaspoon nutmeg
½ teaspoon oregano
2 teaspoons salt

Preheat oven to 350°.

To prepare cream sauce: Place butter in top of double boiler over hot water. Add egg yolks one at a time. Beat constantly with rotary or hand electric beater. Add ¼ cup water, cream, and, Parmesan cheese. Continue to beat until sauce thickens, about 7 to 10 minutes.

Pare and slice eggplant. Sprinkle salt on slices. Place colander on a large plate, arrange eggplant in colander, and cover with another large plate. Let drain for ½ hour, then dry each slice with a paper towel.

Heat 2 tablespoons olive oil in a large skillet. Add onion and green pepper. Sauté until light brown. Add garlic and meat. Sauté until brown.

Add tomato sauce, 1 cup water, cumin, nutmeg, oregano, and salt. Simmer for 15 minutes.

Heat remaining 4 tablespoons of olive oil, and sauté eggplant slices until lightly brown. Drain on paper towels.

Place half the eggplant slices in a well-oiled baking dish. Spread with half the meat mixture. Place remaining eggplant slices on top and cover with the rest of the meat.

Cover the top with cream sauce.

Bake for 30 minutes.

Makes 6 servings.

6.6 GRAMS PER SERVING

Calves Liver in Red Wine

1 pound calves liver, sliced
6 shallots, finely chopped
½ pint dry red wine
Juice of 1 lemon
4 tablespoons oil

½ teaspoon oregano
½ teaspoon seasoned salt
¼ teaspoon black pepper
4 tablespoons butter

Combine shallots, wine, lemon juice, oil, oregano, salt, and pepper in a large bowl. Marinate the liver for 1 hour, then turn it and marinate for another hour.

Remove liver from the marinate.

Melt butter in a pan, and sauté liver for 5 minutes on each side.

Makes 4 servings.

1.8 GRAMS PER SERVING

Veal Rolls

4 veal cutlets, flattened with
   a mallet
½ teaspoon seasoned salt
4 slices boiled ham
6 slices Swiss cheese

1 egg, beaten
¼ cup grated Parmesan
   cheese
4 tablespoons sweet butter
¼ cup dry white wine

Preheat oven to 350°.

Wash and dry veal. Sprinkle with salt. Place 1 slice of ham and 1 slice of cheese on each cutlet. Roll up and tie with string. Dip rolls in egg and Parmesan cheese.

Melt butter in a heavy pan. Sauté veal rolls until they are brown on all sides.

Remove rolls to a small baking dish. Pour sauce from pan and wine over rolls. Top with 2 remaining slices of cheese.

Bake for ½ hour. Remove string and serve.
Makes 4 servings.

Note: This may be used as an hors d'oeuvre by cutting the rolls into pieces the size of half dollars.

1.0 GRAM PER SERVING

Vegetables

Celery and Almonds

2 tablespoons butter
½ cup blanched almonds
4 cups celery, sliced in
    ½-inch pieces
1 chicken bouillon cube,
    crushed

2 tablespoons minced onion
1 packet sugar substitute
⅛ teaspoon garlic powder
⅛ teaspoon ground ginger
⅛ teaspoon ground nutmeg

Melt the butter in a skillet. Add the almonds and sauté on a low flame until lightly browned.

Add the celery, bouillon cube, onion, sugar substitute, garlic powder, ginger, and nutmeg. Stir well. Cook for 10 minutes uncovered, until slightly tender but still crisp.

Makes 4 servings.

8 GRAMS PER SERVING

Eggplant Parmigiana

1 large eggplant, cut into ½-
    inch slices
4 tablespoons olive oil
1 large onion, chopped
2 cloves garlic, minced
1 pound ground chuck
1 8-ounce can tomato sauce

1 cup water
1 teaspoon oregano
½ cup grated Parmesan
    cheese
1 8-ounce package Mozza-
    rella cheese, sliced

Soak eggplant in salted water for 1 hour. Dry with paper towels.

Preheat oven to 350°.

Heat 2 tablespoons olive oil in a skillet and lightly brown the chopped onion. Add garlic and sauté one more minute.

Add ground chuck, stir and cook. When the meat turns brown, add tomato sauce and water. Simmer for 15 minutes.

Place the remaining olive oil in a large skillet on medium heat, and sauté a few eggplant slices at a time until golden brown; add a little more oil if needed.

Oil a baking dish and arrange half of the eggplant slices on the bottom. Cover with half the tomato mixture. Sprinkle with half of the Parmesan cheese and half of the Mozzarella. Repeat these layers.

Bake for 25 to 30 minutes until golden brown.

Makes 8 servings.

6.7 GRAMS PER SERVING

Fried Eggplant

1 medium eggplant	1 cup Hi-Protein bread
1 egg	crumbs
1½ teaspoons salt	4 tablespoons olive oil
¼ teaspoon pepper	Grated Parmesian cheese

Wash the eggplant; pare and cut into finger-length strips.

Beat the egg in a small bowl, add salt and pepper.

Dip eggplant in egg, then roll in bread crumbs.

Heat the oil in a large skillet on medium heat, and sauté eggplant until brown. Sprinkle with Parmesan cheese.

Makes 6 servings.

6.7 GRAMS PER SERVING

Fried Zucchini

Slice 3 zucchini into long, thin strips, discarding seedy centers.

Follow the recipe for fried eggplant.
Makes 6 servings.

6.0 GRAMS PER SERVING

Spicy Eggplant

1 eggplant, pared, sliced ¼-inch thick	Paprika
	¼ cup soya flour
Prepared mustard	¼ - ½ cup oil
Onion salt	

Cut eggplant slices in half. Spread one side very lightly with mustard, sprinkle with onion salt and paprika, and dip both sides very lightly in flour. Heat oil to sizzling, and add eggplant slices, mustard side down. Lower flame and cook on other side until golden brown. Drain and serve hot.
Makes 6 servings.

6.4 GRAMS PER SERVING

Mushroom and Celery Sauté

1 pound fresh mushrooms,
    stems removed
4 cups sliced celery
¾ cup dry white wine
¼ cup lemon juice
¼ cup butter, melted
¼ teaspoon onion powder

¼ teaspoon pepper
1 teaspoon salt
1 tablespoon arrowroot flour,
    dissolved in 1 tablespoon
    cold water
⅛ teaspoon thyme
1 tablespoon chopped parsley

Preheat oven to 375°.

Wash mushrooms and place a layer in a lightly greased ovenproof dish. Add a layer of celery. Mix together all remaining ingredients except parsley. Pour half over mushroom-celery mixture. Place remaining mushrooms, then celery, over mixture. Pour remaining sauce over dish. Top with sprinkled parsley. Bake for 1 hour.

Makes 6 servings.

0.8 GRAM PER SERVING

Seasoned Spinach

1 tablespoon olive oil
1 tablespoon butter
2 packages frozen spinach,
    or 20 ounces fresh,
    steamed, and drained
1 clove garlic, minced

1 teaspoon salt
¼ teaspoon crushed marjoram
3 tablespoons dry Vermouth
Grated Parmesan cheese

Heat oil and butter in skillet. Add all other ingredients except cheese, and blend together. Cook, covered, for 10 minutes over low flame. Sprinkle with grated cheese and serve.

Makes 6 servings.

3.2 GRAMS PER SERVING

Baked Tomatoes and Cheese

5 large firm tomatoes
½ cup grated Parmesan
    cheese
¼ teaspoon oregano
Pinch salt and pepper

1 teaspoon parsley flakes
2 small onions, grated
2 tablespoons butter, melted
1 tablespoon wheat germ
2 tablespoons olive oil

Preheat oven to 350°.

Wash, peel, and slice tomatoes in ½-inch slices. Mix cheese, oregano, salt, pepper, and parsley. Brown onion in butter, add spices, stirring well, and spread on tomato slices. Sprinkle tops with wheat germ and oil.

Place slices carefully on greased cookie sheet or shallow rectangular pan. Bake about 4 or 5 minutes, until cooked through and golden brown.

Makes 6 servings.

5.9 GRAMS PER SERVING

Zucchini Milano

3 medium zucchini
¼ cup olive oil
2 tablespoons wine vinegar
¼ teaspoon oregano

¼ teaspoon basil
½ teaspoon salt
3 tablespoons grated Parme-
    san cheese

Slice zucchini, leaving skin on. Place in a skillet with olive oil, vinegar, oregano, basil, and salt.

Simmer for 8 to 10 minutes.

Turn zucchini carefully with a spatula.

Sprinkle with Parmesan cheese. Cover. Simmer for 10 minutes or until tender.

Makes 4 servings.

4.5 GRAMS PER SERVING

Salads

Bean Sprout Salad

2 pounds canned bean
    sprouts, or fresh if
    possible
1 clove garlic, minced
¼ cup soy sauce
2 tablespoons wine vinegar
2 tablespoons sesame seed
    oil

1 teaspoon honey
1 tablespoon canned
    pimiento strips
3 tablespoons chopped
    scallion
¼ teaspoon black pepper

Combine bean sprouts and cold water and soak for 1 minute. Drain.

Blend rest of ingredients except pimientos, scallion, and pepper. Pour dressing over bean sprouts, and toss with pimiento and scallion.

Season with pepper and serve.
Makes 4 servings.

5.4 GRAMS PER SERVING

Marinated Bean Salad

2 cups cooked green beans
1 small onion, chopped
½ cup Italian Dressing
    1 or 2 (page 111)

1 cup bean sprouts
    (optional)

Combine all ingredients. Chill 1 hour or overnight. Serve on lettuce leaves.

Makes 6 servings.

6.8 GRAMS PER SERVING

Frozen Berry and Nut Salad

1 package D-zerta straw-
    berry gelatin
Pinch salt
1½ cups boiling water
1 tablespoon lemon-juice
4 packets sugar substitute
1 tablespoon Strawberry
    liqueur or diet straw-
    berry syrup

1 teaspoon strawberry
    extract
¼ cup mayonnaise
1 package frozen straw-
    berries (unsweetened) or
    8 ounces fresh, cooked
    strawberries
½ cup chopped walnuts
1¼ cups heavy cream,
    whipped

Dissolve gelatin and salt in boiling water. Stir in lemon juice, sugar substitute, and strawberry flavorings. Blend in mayonnaise. Chill until very thick.

Fold strawberries, nuts, and whipped cream into gelatin mixture. Pour into 9 × 5 × 3-inch loaf pan and freeze until very firm, about 6 hours.

Slice to serve.

Makes 8 servings.

6.3 GRAMS PER SERVING

Crunchy Seafood Salad

1 6 ½-ounce can tuna fish
1 6-ounce can crabmeat
1 5-ounce can shrimp
1 large head lettuce
1 cup diced celery
½ cup diced green onions
½ medium ripe avocado, diced

½ cup chopped walnuts
½ cup roasted unsalted soybeans
½ cup sunflower seeds
2 hard-boiled eggs, diced
1 tomato cut in wedges

Drain the 3 cans of seafood, discard bony tissue from crab, and remove vein down the back of shrimp. Place in a bowl and refrigerate.

Combine remaining ingredients except tomato, in a large salad bowl, and toss well.

Add seafood and toss again.

Add salad dressing of your choice.

Toss again before serving, and decorate with tomato wedges.

Makes 10 servings.

7.7 GRAMS PER SERVING

Spinach Salad

2 cups spinach, washed, dried, and shredded
6 bacon slices, cooked and crumbled

½ cup thinly sliced mushrooms
2 hard-boiled eggs, sliced

Combine all ingredients and serve with Avocado Dressing (page 234).

Makes 4 servings.

5.7 GRAMS PER SERVING

Greek Tarama Salad

Most people are familiar with black and red caviar. The Greeks have a word for another kind of caviar and it is tarama. It makes an excellent salad accompaniment or appetizer.

3 tablespoons tarama (carp roe)	Head of lettuce
1 teaspoon garlic	2 green peppers, sliced
3 tablespoons lemon juice	2 tomatoes, sliced
3 slices Hi-Protein bread	1 cucumber, sliced
¾ cup olive oil	

Place the tarama, garlic, and lemon juice in the small bowl of an electric mixer. Blend on low speed until thoroughly mixed.

Trim crusts from the bread and soak in cold water. Break the bread into the mixture and blend at medium high speed until thoroughly blended. Add oil drop by drop. The mixture should thicken to the consistency of thick mayonnaise.

Serve in the center of a salad tray, ringed with lettuce, peppers, tomatoes, and cucumber.

Makes 8 servings.

Note: Tarama is available in many Greek or Italian stores.

5.8 GRAMS PER SERVING

Sauces, Dressings, Butters, and Jams

Hot Barbecue Sauce

2 tablespoons butter
1 medium onion, chopped
1 clove garlic, minced
¼ cup tomato sauce
2 tablespoons wine vinegar
¼ - ½ teaspoon Tabasco

3 packets sugar substitute
  (brown, if possible)
1 teaspoon salt
1 teaspoon dry mustard
¼ cup water

Melt butter in saucepan. Sauté onion and garlic until golden.
Add remaining ingredients and bring to boil.
  Store in covered jar and refrigerate.
  Makes 1¼ cups.

TOTAL GRAMS 11.5

Lemon Barbecue Sauce

1 small clove garlic
½ teaspoon salt
¼ cup oil
¼ cup lemon juice

2 tablespoons chopped onion
½ teaspoon thyme
1 packet sugar substitute

Mash garlic clove in bowl. Add salt. Dissolve in oil and add
remaining ingredients.
  Chill to blend.

Excellent on grilled fish.
Makes ¾ cup.

TOTAL GRAMS 6.7

Cream Sauce

½ cup mayonnaise
½ cup water
1 tablespoon lemon juice

½ teaspoon seasoned salt
⅛ teaspoon pepper

Combine all ingredients in the top of a double boiler. Stir until smooth and creamy, about 5 minutes.

You can add different herbs to this recipe: basil, thyme, parsley, chopped chives, or celery seed.

TOTAL GRAMS 3.6

Green Sauce

Small bunch fresh basil
      leaves, or 4 tablespoons
      dried basil soaked in oil
      to soften

½ cup grated Parmesan
      cheese
6 cloves garlic, minced
½ cup olive oil
1 tablespoon melted butter

Reduce basil leaves, cheese, and garlic to a smooth paste using a mortar and pestle or a food processor.

Blend in olive oil and butter gradually until thick and creamy sauce is formed.

Makes 1 cup.

TOTAL GRAMS 7.4

"a la King" Sauce

2 tablespoons butter
½ green pepper, chopped
4-ounce can sliced mush-
    rooms
1 tablespoon arrowroot flour
⅓ cup mushroom can liquid

⅓ cup chicken bouillon
⅓ cup heavy cream
½ teaspoon salt
¼ teaspoon paprika
1 teaspoon onion juice
1 pimiento pod, chopped

Heat butter in top of double boiler. Add green pepper and mushrooms and brown directly over flame. Remove from stove, add arrowroot flour, and stir until smooth.

Bring water to a boil in bottom of a double boiler. Add remaining ingredients, except pimiento, to top of double boiler and place over boiling water. Bring contents to boil, stirring constantly.

TOTAL GRAMS 16.8

Chicken "a la King"

Add 2 cups diced cooked chicken and 1 tablespoon Sherry wine.

Makes 4 servings.

TOTAL GRAMS 18.0

Salmon or Tuna "a la King"

Add 1 pound can of salmon or two 7-ounce cans of tuna, drained, and 1 tablespoon Marsala wine.

Makes 4 servings.

TOTAL GRAMS 18.0
2.6 GRAMS PER SERVING

Horseradish Sauce

½ cup sour cream
1 tablespoon prepared horseradish

1 tablespoon grated lemon
  peel
1 teaspoon celery seed
½ teaspoon seasoned salt

Combine all ingredients. Blend well.
  Use with fish or vegetables.

TOTAL GRAMS 7.5

Pasta Sauce, White

3 eggs
2 cups heavy cream

½ cup grated Parmesan
  cheese
Freshly cracked black pepper

Place eggs and cream in the top of a double boiler and whisk
together well. When mixture is about to boil, turn off heat.
Add cheese and pepper. Turn heat back on and simmer for 5
minutes, gently whisking all the time.
  Makes 2½ cups.

TOTAL GRAMS 17.5

SAUCES FOR MEATS, FISH, AND VEGETABLES

Basic White Sauce

Thin:

1 cup heavy cream
¼ tablespoon butter

¼ tablespoon arrowroot
    flour
¼ teaspoon salt

TOTAL GRAMS 9.0

Medium:

1 cup heavy cream
1 tablespoon butter

1 tablespoon arrowroot flour
¼ teaspoon salt

TOTAL GRAMS 11.0

Thick:

1 cup heavy cream
2 tablespoons butter

2 tablespoons arrowroot
    flour
¼ teaspoon salt

TOTAL GRAMS 15.0

Melt butter in a saucepan and blend in flour and salt. Remove from heat. Add cold milk gradually, blending after each addition until smooth. Stir over low heat until thickened.

VARIATIONS:

Horseradish: Add 4 tablespoons well-drained prepared white horseradish to each cup thick white sauce.

TOTAL GRAMS 20.2

Onion: Cook 1 tablespoon grated onion in measured butter of medium white sauce about 2 minutes before adding flour.

TOTAL GRAMS 17.2

Mustard: Add 2 tablespoons prepared mustard, 1 teaspoon grated onion, and 1 teaspoon paprika to each cup medium white sauce.

TOTAL GRAMS 18.0

Cheese: Add 1 cup grated Cheddar cheese and ½ teaspoon Worcestershire sauce to each cup medium white sauce. Stir over very low heat until cheese melts.

TOTAL GRAMS 20.0

Easy Hollandaise: Just before serving, beat 2 egg yolks, 3 tablespoons melted butter, and 1 tablespoon lemon juice into 1 cup thick white sauce.

TOTAL GRAMS 17.6

Egg: Add 2 hard-boiled eggs, chopped, and 1 tablespoon parsley flakes to each cup of medium white sauce.

TOTAL GRAMS 16.4

Sour Cream Sauce

1 pint sour cream
3 tablespoons heavy cream
2 tablespoons minced fresh
    dill

10 turns of the pepper mill
¼ cup grated Parmesan
    cheese
2 tablespoons pine nuts

Combine all ingredients. Refrigerate.
   Use on pasta, vegetables, or as a sauce for meat.
   Makes 2½ cups.

TOTAL GRAMS 26.1

Apricot or Peach Glaze

1 jar diet peach or apricot
    jam
2 packets sugar substitute

1 tablespoon lemon juice
¼ teaspoon ground cloves

Combine all ingredients thoroughly. Spread over poultry or
meat and broil. Keep basting with glaze that drips off until
cooked through and golden brown.

TOTAL GRAMS 3.1

Creamy Celery Seed Dressing

½ cup sour cream
½ cup mayonnaise
2 tablespoons tomato sauce

½ teaspoon Worcestershire
    sauce
½ teaspoon celery seed
½ teaspoon seasoned salt

Combine all ingredients in a screw-top jar.
   Shake well. Refrigerate.
   Makes 1¼ cups.

                                        TOTAL GRAMS 9.8

Curry Dressing

4 tablespoons tarragon vine-   1 tablespoon sour cream
   gar   ¼ teaspoon garlic powder
2 tablespoons olive oil   1 teaspoon sesame seeds
6 tablespoons safflower oil   ½ teaspoon seasoned salt
1 teaspoon lemon juice   1 egg
½ teaspoon curry

Place all ingredients in a screw-top jar. Shake well. Refrigerate.

                                        TOTAL GRAMS 5.3

Dill Vinaigrette Dressing

4 tablespoons tarragon vine-   1 teaspoon lemon juice
   gar   ¼ teaspoon garlic powder
2 tablespoons olive oil   2 teaspoons dry dill or 2 ta-
6 tablespoons safflower oil   blespoons fresh dill
2 tablespoons chopped olives   ½ packet sugar substitute
¼ teaspoon dry mustard   1 egg
1 teaspoon Dijon mustard

Place all ingredients in a screw-top jar. Shake well. Refrigerate.
   Makes 1 cup.

                                        TOTAL GRAMS 4.4

Italian Dressing 1

½ cup olive oil
¼ cup wine vinegar
1 clove garlic, minced

½ teaspoon seasoned salt
¼ teaspoon pepper

Combine all ingredients in a screw-top jar.
  Shake well. Refrigerate.
  Shake again before serving.

TOTAL GRAMS 3.3

Italian Dressing 2

½ cup olive oil
¼ cup wine vinegar
1 clove garlic, minced

¼ teaspoon oregano
½ teaspoon seasoned salt
Dash pepper

Combine all ingredients in a screw-top jar.
  Shake well. Refrigerate.
  Shake again before serving.

TOTAL GRAMS 3.8

Parmesan Caesar Dressing

4 tablespoons tarragon vinegar
2 tablespoons olive oil
6 tablespoons safflower oil
1 teaspoon lemon juice
¼ teaspoon dry mustard
2 teaspoons Dijon mustard

1 tablespoon grated Parmesan cheese
¼ teaspoon garlic powder
1 teaspoon seasoned salt
½ packet sugar substitute
1 egg

Place all ingredients in a screw-top jar. Shake well. Refrigerate.

TOTAL GRAMS 4.6

Sour Cream Mayonnaise Dressing

½ cup mayonnaise
½ cup sour cream
1 teaspoon honey
½ teaspoon mustard

1 tablespoon lemon juice
1 clove garlic mashed
   (optional)

Combine all ingredients in a screw-top jar. Refrigerate.
  Makes 1¼ cups.

TOTAL GRAMS 12.7

Tarragon Dressing

4 tablespoons tarragon
   vinegar
2 tablespoons olive oil
6 tablespoons safflower oil
¼ teaspoon dry mustard
1 teaspoon Dijon mustard

1 teaspoon lemon juice
1 teaspoon tarragon
⅛ teaspoon thyme
¼ teaspoon garlic powder
½ packet sugar substitute
1 egg

Place all ingredients in a screw-top jar. Shake well. Refrigerate.

TOTAL GRAMS 2.9

Garlic Butter

½ cup butter, softened   ½ teaspoon oregano or basil
1 clove garlic, minced

Blend butter, garlic, and oregano or basil in a small bowl.
Makes ½ cup butter.

TOTAL GRAM 0.5

Parsley Butter

½ cup butter   ¼ teaspoon seasoned salt
3 tablespoons lemon juice   Dash paprika
1 tablespoon parsley

Blend ingredients well. Serve with fish, chicken, or veal.

TOTAL GRAMS 3.8

Berry Jam

1 tablespoon sugar-free gela-   ½ cup raspberries
   tin   ½ cup blueberries
1 cup water   Juice of ½ lime
½ cup strawberries   1 packet sugar substitute

Add gelatin to cold water. Bring to boil, stirring until completely dissolved.

Cool gelatin in refrigerator until it reaches consistency of
egg white.

Heat berries in saucepan for about 5 minutes, or until tender. Remove from heat, and crush berries with a fork. Stir for 2 minutes to cool.

Add lime juice and sugar substitute to berries. Stir well. Fold berries into thickened gelatin. Mix well. Refrigerate until jellied.

Makes 2 cups.

TOTAL GRAMS 44.4

The Best Marmalade

4 oranges	2 tablespoons Cointreau
2 lemons	2 teaspoons cinnamon
1 grapefruit	3 packets sugar substitute
2 cups cold water	

Slice oranges, lemons, and grapefruit into very thin slices. Place in a saucepan, add water, cover, and boil gently for 2 hours. Uncover, add Cointreau, and simmer for 1 hour more. Cool; add cinnamon and sugar substitute. Refrigerate.

Makes 4 cups.

44.4 GRAMS PER CUP

Breads

———◆———

Hi-Protein Soya Bread

3 eggs
2 tablespoons sour cream
2 tablespoons butter, melted

½ cup soya flour
1 teaspoon baking powder
½ teaspoon baking soda

Preheat oven to 325°.

Mix eggs, sour cream, and butter in a bowl. Add soya flour, baking powder, and baking soda. Beat well until smooth.

Place in a well-greased 8½ x 4½ x 2½-inch loaf pan. Bake 45 to 50 minutes.

Makes 12 slices.

TOTAL GRAMS 35.5
2.9 GRAMS PER SLICE

Nut Muffins

Follow preceding recipe adding ½ cup chopped nuts. Place in well-greased muffin tins and bake for 35-45 minutes.

Makes 6 muffins.

7.5 GRAMS PER MUFFIN

Rye Bread

Follow preceding recipe adding 1 tablespoon caraway seeds. Place in well-greased tin and bake for 45 to 50 minutes.
   Makes 12 slices.

3.1 GRAMS PER SLICE

Peanut Butter Muffins

Follow preceding recipe adding 2 tablespoons peanut butter. Place in well greased muffin tins and bake 35 to 45 minutes. minutes.
   Makes 6 muffins.

6.0 GRAMS PER MUFFIN

Croutons

1 cup Hi-Protein soya bread,   2 tablespoons butter
     cut into ½-inch cubes

Heat butter in a skillet. Add bread, stir carefully until toasted.
   You may sprinkle with garlic salt, seasoned salt, or onion salt. Or add 1 tablespoon minced onion and herbs.

TOTAL GRAMS 32

Desserts

———◆———

Basic Crepe

3 eggs
½ cup soya powder
½ cup heavy cream

1 tablespoon wheat germ
1 teaspoon safflower oil

Place all ingredients in a blender. Blend until smooth.
Makes 16 crepes.

2.9 GRAMS PER CREPE

Dessert Crepes

3 eggs
½ cup soya powder
½ cup heavy cream
1 tablespoon wheat germ

1 teaspoon safflower oil
2 packets sugar substitute
1 teaspoon Crème de Cacao

Place all ingredients in a blender. Blend until smooth.
Makes 16 crepes.

3.0 GRAMS PER CREPE

Cottage Cheese Dessert Salad

2 envelopes unflavored gelatin
½ cup cold water
2 cups creamed cottage cheese
1 cup mayonnaise
1 cup heavy cream
1 tablespoon lemon juice
Dash Tabasco

1 packet sugar substitute
Pinch salt
1 teaspoon vanilla
1 cup mixed berries, marinated in 2 tablespoons fruit liqueur and 2 packets brown sugar substitute

Sprinkle gelatin on cold water in top of double boiler, and cool slightly. Combine cottage cheese and mayonnaise and stir into gelatin.

Whip the cream, and fold into lemon juice, Tabasco, sugar substitute, salt, and vanilla. Spoon into 5-cup ring mold and chill until very firm, 5-6 hours.

Drain berries and set the marinade aside for Yogurt Cream Sauce.

Unmold, and fill the center with drained berries. Serve with Yogurt Cream Sauce.

Yogurt Cream Sauce

½ cup yogurt
½ cup sour cream

2 tablespoons berry liqueur marinade

Mix well and spoon over dessert salad.
Makes 10 servings.

6.4 GRAMS PER SERVING

Almond Custard

1½ cups light cream
4 egg yolks
4 packets sugar substitute

Pinch of seasoned salt
¼ cup chopped almonds

In the top of a double boiler combine the cream, egg yolks, 3 packets sugar substitute, and salt, and cook over simmering water, stirring mixture until it thickens and coats the spoon.

Strain the custard into a serving bowl and let it cool.

Chill the custard, covered, for at least 3 hours.

Combine the almonds with 1 packet sugar substitute and sprinkle over custard before serving.

Makes 4 servings.

3.1 GRAMS PER SERVING

Confetti Mold

1 package diet strawberry gelatin
1 package diet lime gelatin
1 package diet orange gelatin

3 packages diet lemon gelatin
1 cup heavy cream
1 teaspoon vanilla extract

Prepare first 3 diet gelatins separately, using 1½ cups water each. Refrigerate each in separate shallow pans until *thoroughly* firm. Dice each into tiny cubes.

Prepare all lemon diet gelatins using 2¾ cups water. Allow to thicken. When mixture is very thick, but not firm, add heavy cream. Thicken again. Fold in all flavors of gelatin cubes and vanilla extract. Chill until thoroughly firm.

Makes 8 servings.

1.0 GRAM PER SERVING

Chocolate Peanut Butter Cookies

¾ cup soya flour
2 tablespoons cocoa
1½ teaspoons baking powder
4 packets sugar substitute
Pinch salt
⅓ cup peanut butter

1 egg, beaten
1 teaspoon melted butter
½ cup heavy cream
1 teaspoon vanilla extract
½ teaspoon chocolate
    extract

Preheat oven to 400°.
  Sift dry ingredients into bowl.
  Combine peanut butter with remaining ingredients and add to flour mixture. Stir until blended.
  Drop by teaspoon onto greased cookie sheet.
  Bake for 10-12 minutes until brown.
  Makes 24 cookies.

3.2 GRAMS PER COOKIE

Spice Cookies

1 tablespoon wheat germ
½ cup soya flour
¼ cup ground almonds
1 packet sugar substitute

⅓ cup butter, chilled
Pinch cinnamon
Pinch nutmeg
2 egg whites, beaten

Mix together first 4 ingredients. Cut up butter and work into dry ingredients. Sprinkle with spices and fold in whites.
  Drop by spoonfuls on a cookie sheet, spacing 1½ inches apart. Bake for 12 to 15 minutes.
  Makes 1 dozen cookies.

2.4 GRAMS PER COOKIE

Lemon Sponge Cake

½ cup cream
1 cup soya flour
1½ teaspoons baking powder
Dash salt

3 eggs
8 packets sugar substitute
2 teaspoons vanilla
1 teaspoon lemon extract

Preheat oven to 300°.

Scald cream and remove from heat.

Sift flour, baking powder, and salt together.

Beat eggs and sugar substitute thoroughly until thick and lemon colored. Blend in flour mixture just until smooth. Add warm cream and extracts to mixture. Pour batter immediately into a 9-inch greased tube pan. Bake for 30 minutes.

Makes 8 servings.

TOTAL GRAMS 32.19
4.5 GRAMS PER SERVING

Light Sponge Cake

7 eggs, separated
¾ teaspoon cream of tartar
Pinch salt
½ cup water

8 packets sugar substitute
1 teaspoon anise extract
1 teaspoon vanilla extract
1 cup soya flour

Preheat oven to 300°.

Beat egg whites until foamy. Add cream of tartar and beat until stiff peaks form.

Beat yolks until thick. Add salt, water, sugar substitute, and extracts. Fold in flour. Stir both mixtures lightly together until no lumps appear.

Immediately place in greased tube pan in oven. Bake for **1** hour.

Makes 8 servings.

TOTAL GRAMS 23.0
2.8 GRAMS PER SERVING

Sponge Torte

⅓ cup soya flour
½ teaspoon baking powder
Pinch salt
2 eggs

8 packets sugar substitute
1 teaspoon vanilla extract
½ teaspoon almond extract

Preheat oven to 325°.

Sift flour, baking powder, and salt together.

Beat eggs and sugar substitute thoroughly until thick and lemon-colored. Stir in extracts. Fold in flour mixture. Bake in a greased 8-inch layer pan for 30 minutes.

Makes 8 servings.

TOTAL GRAMS 25.6
3.2 GRAMS PER SERVING

Spice Cake

½ cup cream
1 cup soya flour
1½ teaspoons baking powder
Pinch salt
½ teaspoon cinnamon
⅛ teaspoon ground cloves

¼ teaspoon nutmeg
3 eggs
8 packets sugar substitute
1 teaspoon brandy extract
2 teaspoons vanilla extract

Preheat oven to 325°.

Scald cream and remove from heat. Sift flour, baking powder, salt, and spices together.

Beat eggs with sugar substitute until *very* thick. Blend in flour mixture until smooth. Add warm cream and extracts to mixture. Pour batter immediately into 8-inch greased layer pan.

Bake for 30 minutes.

Makes 8 servings.

TOTAL GRAMS 34.5
4.6 GRAMS PER SERVING

Chocolate Sponge Layer Cake

½ cup soya flour
½ teaspoon baking powder
Pinch salt
1 tablespoon unsweetened cocoa

2 eggs
8 packets sugar substitute
1 teaspoon vanilla extract
1 teaspoon diet chocolate extract

Preheat oven to 325°.

Sift flour, baking powder, salt, and cocoa together.

Beat eggs with sugar substitute until *very* thick. Stir in extracts. Fold in flour mixture. Bake in 8-inch greased layer pan for 30 minutes. Makes 1 layer.

Makes 8 servings.

2.4 GRAMS PER SERVING

Lemon Cake Custard Pudding

¼ cup soya flour, sifted
Pinch salt
10 packets sugar substitute
3 egg yolks, beaten
1½ cups scalded cream
1 teaspoon vanilla

1 teaspoon lemon extract
2 tablespoons oil
2 tablespoons lemon juice
1 teaspoon grated lemon rind
3 egg whites, stiffly beaten

Preheat oven to 325°.

Sift dry ingredients. Combine yolks, cream, flavorings, oil, lemon juice, and rind. Add to flour mixture. Fold in egg whites.

Pour into 8 greased, ovenproof custard cups. Bake for 45 minutes to 1 hour. Serve cold.

Makes 8 servings.

4.0 GRAMS PER SERVING

Pie Crust I

¼ cup butter, cut in pieces   Pinch salt
½ cup water   2 eggs
1 cup soya flour

Preheat oven to 425°.

Boil water in saucepan. Add cut-up pieces of butter to boiling water and stir to dissolve. Add flour and salt; mix well. Lower heat to simmer. Stir until no lumps remain. Remove from heat. Add eggs and mix thoroughly.

Cover with waxed paper and refrigerate for about 1 hour.

Place in pie pan by tablespoons, patting sides and bottom with back of spoon. Use fork tines to decorate edges of piecrust, and to prick holes in bottom and sides of crust.

Arrange empty disposable pie plate over pie (to keep crust from puffing). Bake for 30 minutes until solid and brown around edges. Remove second pan, cover edges with foil, and allow center to brown thoroughly. Cool.

TOTAL GRAMS 34.2

Pumpkin Ice Cream

2 cups cooked pumpkin,
    fresh or canned
5 eggs
2 cups heavy cream
1 teaspoon vanilla

1 teaspoon cinnamon
¼ teaspoon nutmeg
⅛ teaspoon allspice
6 packets sugar substitute

Combine all ingredients in blender until smooth. Freeze. Stir occasionally until frozen.
    Makes 8 servings.

6.4 GRAMS PER SERVING

Cranberry Frost

1 pound fresh cranberries
4 cups water
8 packets sugar substitute
1 teaspoon orange extract

1 tablespoon Cranberry
    liqueur (optional)
1 package diet orange gelatin

Cook cranberries in water over low flame until skins pop. Strain through sieve and heat. Remove from stove, and add sugar substitute, flavorings, and gelatin. Stir until totally dissolved.

Chill until cold, stir, and pour into freezer trays. Freeze about 2 hours, then beat well and return to trays.

Freeze until firm, about 3 hours.
    Makes 8 servings.

6.2 GRAMS PER SERVING

Peanut Butter Ice Cream

6 eggs, separated
1 teaspoon vanilla
6 packets sugar substitute

3 tablespoons chunky peanut butter
½ pint heavy cream

Beat egg yolks, vanilla, and 3 packets sugar substitute until light. Stir in peanut butter until smooth.

Whip cream with remaining sugar substitute. Fold whipped cream into peanut butter mixture.

Beat egg whites until stiff peaks form and fold into mixture. Pour into freezer trays, cover with transparent wrap, and freeze until firm. Or pour into your ice cream maker.

If ice cream has been in the freezer for more than 6 hours before serving, allow to stand at room temperature for 15 minutes.

Makes 6 servings.

3.3 GRAMS PER SERVING

Almond Coconut Candies

1 8-ounce package cream cheese
1 tablespoon heavy cream
½ teaspoon almond extract
½ teaspoon coconut extract

1 packet sugar substitute
¼ cup ground almonds
½ cup shredded un-sweetened coconut

Soften cheese with cream. Add extracts, sugar substitute and almonds. Roll into 1-inch balls and coat with coconut. Chill.

Makes 24 candies.

3.0 GRAMS PER CANDY

Coconut Candy

3-ounce package cream
    cheese
½ cup chopped apples,
    sprinkled with lemon
    juice

½ cup chopped walnuts
1 tablespoon wheat germ
2 teaspoons honey
½ cup unsweetened coconut

Mix all ingredients except coconut until moist.
    Shape into 16 balls, about 1½ inch size. Roll in coconut.
    Store in refrigerator.
    Makes 16 candies.

2.7 GRAMS PER CANDY

Marzipan

1 7-ounce package un-
    sweetened coconut,
    finely grated
1 package diet gelatin
    (any fruit flavor)

1 cup ground almonds
½ cup heavy cream
4 packets sugar substitute
½ teaspoon vanilla extract
½ teaspoon almond extract

Combine all ingredients. Shape into any designs you like—
fruits, vegetables, etc. (Food coloring may be added to simu-
late true details.)
    Chill until forms hold their shape.
    Makes 2 dozen 1-inch forms.

3.5 GRAMS PER SERVING

Beverages

Hot Coffee Protein Drink

1 cup coffee, very hot
1 tablespoon cottage cheese
½ teaspoon cinnamon

1 teaspoon coffee liqueur
1 envelope sugar substitute
1 teaspoon brewer's yeast

Place all ingredients in a blender. Blend until smooth.
Makes 1 serving.

3.8 GRAMS PER SERVING

Coffee-Maple Breakfast Protein

1 cup brewed coffee
1 tablespoon maple extract
2 tablespoon sour cream
1 envelope sugar substitute
2 eggs

1 teaspoon brewer's yeast
1 tablespoon liquid
6 ice cubes
1 tablespoon liquid lecithin

Place all ingredients in a blender. Blend until smooth.
Makes 1 serving.

3.2 GRAMS PER SERVING

Mocha Breakfast Drink

1 cup brewed coffee
1 cup diet chocolate soda
1 tablespoon diet chocolate
    syrup
4 ice cubes
¼ teaspoon cinnamon

2 tablespoons heavy cream
1 teaspoon brewer's yeast
1 egg
Sugar substitute to taste
    (optional)

Place all ingredients in a blender and blend until smooth.
  Makes 1 serving.

4.0 GRAMS PER SERVING

Spiced Iced Coffee

2 tablespoons instant coffee
5 whole allspice
5 whole cloves
Dash cinnamon

3 cups boiling water
8 ice cubes
4 teaspoons cream

Combine all ingredients except cream in a 1-quart container.
  Cover and refrigerate 1 hour or more.
  Strain. Pour over ice cubes into 4 tall glasses.
  Add 1 teaspoon cream to each glass.
  Makes 4 servings.

0.3 GRAM PER SERVING

Black Cow

¾ glass diet root beer
1 tablespoon cream

Ice cubes

Combine all ingredients in a tall glass.
  Makes 1 serving.

0.4 GRAM PER SERVING

Cola Cow

Follow preceding recipe using diet cola, or a scoop of diet ice cream instead of cream.

3.6 GRAMS PER SERVING

Cool Lime Mint with Lecithin

2 cups warm water
½ cup lime juice
⅛ teaspoon mint extract
1 packet sugar substitute

1 tablespoon lecithin granules
1 pint diet lime soda

Combine water, lime juice, and mint extract; chill for 2 hours or more in refrigerator.

Add sugar substitute, lecithin, and soda to chilled lime mixture.

Pour into glasses with 2 ice cubes. Garnish with lime slices and a sprig of fresh mint.

Makes 4 servings.

2.5 GRAMS PER SERVING

Brewer's Yeast Hibiscus Drink

1 cup hibiscus tea (available
  in specialty and health
  food stores)
2 tablespoons heavy cream
1 packet sugar substitute

2 teaspoons artificially
  sweetened raspberry
  syrup
1 teaspoon brewer's yeast
3 ice cubes

Place all ingredients in blender. Blend well.

Makes 1 serving.

2.6 GRAMS PER SERVING

DIET 2

MENU PLAN
FOR DIET 2

———◆———

DAY ONE

Breakfast:

Boursin and Lecithin Omelet
Two slices ham
One slice whole wheat bread
Coffee

Lunch:

Avocado Cottage Cheese Mold
One Orange Pecan Muffin
Diet soda

Dinner:

Bran-Nut Chicken
Sweet Baked Lentils
Green Beans au Gratin
Green salad with two tablespoons Thousand
Island Dressing
One Special Brownie
Coffee

DAY TWO

Breakfast:

Two slices French Toast
4 strips bacon
Coffee

Lunch:

Spicy Chicken
Green salad with two tablespoons Dill-Vinaigrette
Dressing
Pumpkin Custard
Tea

Dinner:

Curried Tuna Rice Salad
Apple Cabbage
Poppy Seed Cake
Coffee

DAY THREE

Breakfast:

Basic Omelet
   Two tablespoons Blueberry Jam
      Two strips bacon
         One slice Zucchini Bread
            Coffee

Lunch:

Couscous and Tuna Stuffed Pepper
   Strawberry Cheese Pudding
      Diet soda

Dinner:

Meat Loaf with Grains or Cereal
   Special Squash
      Green salad with 2 tablespoons Yogurt Dressing
         Baked Brown Rice Pudding
            Coffee

DAY FOUR

Breakfast:

Reuben Omelet
   One slice Orange Health Loaf
      Coffee

Lunch:

Peanut and Carrot Salad
   Lemon Chiffon Pie
      Diet soda

Dinner:

Roast chicken
   Soya Couscous Dressing for Poultry
      Wok Vegetables
         Green salad with two tablespoons Avocado
         Dressing
            One Apple Nut Pinwheel
               Coffee

DAY FIVE

Breakfast:

   Blintz Omelet
      Two sausages
         Orange Bran Muffin
            Coffee

Lunch:

   Summertime Bean Salad (with garbanzo beans)
      Half a grapefruit
         Diet soda

Dinner:

   Shrimp and Scallops Mark
      Barley Pilaf
         Carrots and Herbs
            Green salad with two tablespoons Tarragon
            Dressing
               Caramel Cream
                  Coffee

DAY SIX

Breakfast:

Vegetable Omelet
One slice Zucchini Bread
Coffee

Lunch:

Sweet Barley Soup
Orange Pecan Muffin
Tea

Dinner:

Steak au Poivre
Carrot Ring
One cup mixed green salad
with two tablespoons Parmesan Caesar Dressing
Two Pumpkin Nut Cookies
Coffee

DAY SEVEN

Breakfast:

    Creamy Peach Omelet
      One slice whole wheat bread
        Coffee

Lunch:

    Cream of Cauliflower Soup with Soy Flakes
      One orange
        Tea

Dinner:

    Wok Steak 1
      Fried Rice
        Green salad with two tablespoons of Curry
        Dressing
          Two Tahini Cookies
            Coffee

RECIPES
FOR DIET 2

———◆———

Appetizers

Crunchy

½ cup peanuts
½ cup cashews
¼ cup soy flakes
¼ cup pumpkin seeds
¼ cup sunflower seeds

5 tablespoons butter
¼ cup Worcestershire sauce
2 teaspoons chili powder
1 teaspoon garlic salt
½ teaspoon seasoned salt

Preheat oven to 225°.

Combine peanuts, cashews, soy flakes, pumpkin seeds and sunflower seeds in a baking pan.

Heat butter in a pot and add remaining ingredients. Pour over peanut mixture. Mix well. Cover and bake 1 hour.

Remove cover, bake 1 hour longer, stirring occasionally.

Cool and store in a jar with an airtight lid.

TOTAL GRAMS 80.7

Nuts Sweet Nuts

2 tablespoons melted butter
1 egg, beaten
½ cup honey
½ cup bran
½ cup soy flakes
2 teaspoons cinnamon

1 teaspoon allspice
½ cup chopped almonds
½ cup pumpkin seeds
½ cup chopped walnuts
½ cup sunflower seeds

Preheat oven to 300°.

Combine butter, egg, and honey, and blend well. Stir in remaining ingredients.

Spread mixture in a large shallow baking pan. Bake about 20 to 30 minutes until lightly browned. Remove from oven and stir carefully. Spread the nuts and seeds with a fork. Cool.

Store in an airtight jar. Use for snacking.

Makes 4 cups.

50.1 GRAMS PER SERVING

Oriental Snack

½ cup peanuts
½ cup blanched almonds
¼ cup sesame seeds
¼ cup soy flakes
¼ cup rolled oats
¼ cup pumpkin seeds

6 tablespoons butter
¼ cup soy sauce
½ teaspoon onion salt
½ teaspoon seasoned salt
½ teaspoon garlic salt

Preheat oven to 225°.

Combine peanuts, almonds, sesame seeds, soy flakes, rolled oats, and pumpkin seeds in a baking dish.

Heat butter in a pot and add remaining ingredients. Pour over peanut mixture. Mix well. Cover and bake for 1 hour.

Remove cover, bake 1 hour longer, stirring occasionally.

Cool and store in a jar with an airtight lid.

Makes 3½ cups.

TOTAL GRAMS 105.8

Roast Pumpkin Seeds

2 cups pumpkin seeds   1½ teaspoons seasoned salt
2 tablespoons melted butter

Preheat oven to 250°.

Wash and dry pumpkin seeds. In a shallow pan combine seeds, butter, and salt. Mix well. Roast for 30 to 40 minutes, stirring often to brown evenly.

Makes 2 cups.

TOTAL GRAMS 85.5

Soups

Sweet Barley Soup

½ cup barley
3 tablespoons butter
1½ cups carrots, in chunks
1½ cups celery, in chunks
2 large onions, sliced
1 clove garlic, minced

1½ cups butternut squash, cut in chunks
2 tablespoons chopped parsley
2 teaspoons seasoned salt
½ teaspoon pepper
1 teaspoon marjoram

Bring 2 cups water to a boil, add barley, cover and simmer for 40 minutes. Set aside.

Melt butter in a large pot, and sauté carrots, celery, onions, and garlic until golden. Add 1 quart water and remaining ingredients. Cover; simmer until all vegetables are soft, about 20 to 30 minutes.

Place half into blender, blend well, then add and blend the other half.

Place soup back in pot; add barley, heat, and serve.

Makes 4 servings.

38.5 GRAMS PER SERVING

Special Bean Soup

2 cups dried beans
1½ quarts water
1 tablespoon salt
2 tablespoons butter
2 carrots, sliced thin
2 leeks, sliced thin

2 stalks celery
¼ cup chopped onion
¼ pound salt pork
3 bay leaves and 1 teaspoon savory (tied in small cheesecloth bag)

145

Place the dried beans in a saucepan with water to cover. Let them soak for 2 hours, then drain. Add 1½ quarts water and salt, and bring to a boil. Skim well.

Melt the butter in a large skillet. Add the sliced carrots, leeks, celery, and onions, and sauté until golden. Add the beans in their liquid with the piece of salt pork. Add herbs, cover, and cook slowly, adding water if necessary, to keep beans covered.

Remove pork and herbs and rub the mixture through a sieve or puree in blender.

Return to pot and thin slightly with additional water. Heat to simmering.

Makes 8 servings.

16.2 GRAMS PER SERVING

Cream of Cauliflower Soup with Soy Flakes

½ cup raw barley
3 tablespoons butter
1 large onion, chopped
3 stalks celery, chopped
3 medium carrots, chopped
1 clove garlic, minced

1 small cauliflower
⅛ teaspoon nutmeg
Salt and pepper to taste
½ cup soy flakes
½ cup cream

Boil 2 cups water; add barley, cover, and simmer for 35 to 40 minutes until water is absorbed.

Meanwhile, in a large pot melt butter, and add onion, celery, carrots, and garlic. Sauté until golden.

Wash cauliflower; cut off tough end of stem, remove leaves, break into flowerets.

To the sautéed vegetables, add cauliflower, 4 cups water, nutmeg, salt, and pepper. Bring to a boil, cover, simmer for about 12 minutes until cauliflower is tender.

Place soup in a blender, one half at a time, and blend well.

Replace in the pot, add barley, soy flakes, and cream; heat again.

Makes 8 servings.

18.4 GRAMS PER SERVING

Court Bouillon

2 pounds fish trimmings
  from firm white fish
2 quarts water
1 bay leaf
¼ pound butter
2 carrots, diced
3 stalks celery, diced
1 quart dry white wine

7 peppercorns
2 teaspoons salt
2 small onions, minced
⅛ teaspoon thyme
1 teaspoon dried parsley
  flakes or 2 tablespoons
  fresh parsley

Place fish trimmings in deep pot. Add the remaining ingredients and bring to a boil on medium flame. Cover and cook gently for 1 hour.

Remove fish from liquid and strain bouillon.

Use as directed in recipes.

Makes 2 quarts.

TOTAL GRAMS 35.0

Main Dishes

Bran-Nut Chicken

4 pounds of chicken parts
⅓ cup bran
¼ cup melted butter
½ cup honey

¼ cup soy sauce
½ cup sesame seeds
¼ cup slivered almonds

Preheat oven to 350°.

Place chicken in a shallow baking dish. Combine bran, butter, honey, and soy sauce. Pour over chicken.

Bake for 30 minutes. Add sesame seeds and almonds. Bake for 30 minutes more, basting frequently.

Makes 8 servings.

29.7 GRAMS PER SERVING

Spicy Chicken

4 tablespoons butter
3 pounds chicken legs, thighs, or breasts
1 large onion, sliced
3 garlic cloves, minced
1 cup sour cream
2 cups chicken broth
¼ teaspoon ground cardamom
1 mild cherry pepper, seeds removed, chopped

1 teaspoon chopped mint leaves
½ teaspoon cinnamon
½ teaspoon ground ginger
¼ teaspoon ground cloves
1 teaspoon salt
1 tablespoon ground coriander
1 teaspoon turmeric
2 tablespoons lemon juice
1 cup couscous

Preheat oven to 300°.

Heat butter in a skillet. Sauté chicken until golden. Remove chicken.

Sauté onion and garlic in the same pan.

Meanwhile, combine remaining ingredients, except lemon juice and couscous, in a medium bowl. Mix well.

When onion and garlic are light brown, add sour cream mixture.

Add the chicken and sprinkle with lemon juice. Cover and simmer for 15 minutes.

Oil a large baking dish. Spread uncooked couscous on the bottom. Spoon chicken and sauce on top.

Cover tightly and bake for 15 minutes.

Makes 4 servings.

55.8 GRAMS PER SERVING

Meat Loaf with Grains or Cereal

2 large stalks celery, sliced	3 eggs
1 large onion, sliced	1 cup cooked grain, cereal,
3 tablespoons butter	couscous, kasha, millet,
2 cloves garlic, minced	barley, or oats
2 pounds ground beef, pork, or veal	Seasoned salt and pepper

Preheat oven to 350°.

Sauté celery and onion in butter in a skillet until golden brown. Add garlic at the last minute. Place the ground meat in a bowl. Add onion mixture, eggs, grain or cereal, and salt and pepper. Mix well with your hands. Shape into a loaf, and place in a lightly oiled pan. Bake for 1 hour.

Note: You can experiment with this recipe by adding 1 teaspoon oregano, basil, thyme, or curry, or 2 to 4 tablespoons tomato sauce.

Makes 6 servings.

31.5 GRAMS PER SERVING

Wok Steak I

6 tablespoons peanut oil
1 medium onion, sliced
1 large zucchini, cut in half-dollar slices
½ pound snow pea pods
½ pound mushrooms, sliced
½ can water chestnuts

2 tablespoons sesame seeds
1 pound beef fillet or London broil, sliced thin
2 tablespoons Gravy Master
¼ pound bean sprouts
3 tablespoons dark soy sauce

Heat 2 tablespoons of oil in a wok. Add vegetables in order of listing, allowing 1 minute cooking time between each addition. Add sesame seeds and 2 more tablespoons of oil. Toss well.

Sprinkle steak with Gravy Master, mix well. Move vegetables to one side of wok. Add remaining oil in the bottom and place steak in the oil. Cook about 1 minute, turn, and cook 1 minute more. Toss steak with vegetables. Add bean sprouts and soy sauce. Toss well. Serve immediately.

Makes 4 servings.

27.0 GRAMS PER SERVING

Basic Stew

1 pound stewing beef
¼ cup peanut oil
2 tablespoons wheat germ
¼ pound small white onions, peeled and halved
½ small acorn squash, peeled and cubed

10 large mushrooms, halved
2 packets beef broth mix
½ cup dry red wine
½ cup water
2 teaspoons garlic powder
1 tablespoon seasoned salt
¼ pound bean sprouts

Heat oil in large pan.

Roll beef in wheat germ and add to pan with onions, water

chestnuts, squash, and mushrooms. Sprinkle with beef broth mix. Sauté for 7 minutes.

Transfer into a large saucepan. Stir in wine, water, garlic powder, and salt. Cover and allow to simmer for 1 hour. Add bean sprouts. Cook ½ hour longer.

Makes 4 servings.

10.1 GRAMS PER SERVING

Chinese Cabbage with Ham

3 tablespoons peanut oil	½ teaspoon ground ginger
2 pounds white cabbage, rinsed, cored, and coarsely chopped	2 tablespoons sherry
	2 teaspoons soy sauce.
½ teaspoon garlic powder	1 tablespoon gluten powder
¼ pound cooked ham, cut into strips	¼ cup chicken broth
	Salt to taste

Heat the oil in a wok or skillet. Add cabbage and garlic powder and stir-fry the mixture for 3 minutes. Add ham and ginger and cook 1 minute longer.

Mix sherry with soy sauce and stir into cabbage.

Mix gluten powder with chicken broth and stir into cabbage until sauce is thickened and cabbage is well coated.

Add salt to taste and serve immediately.

Makes 4 servings.

11 GRAMS PER SERVING

Couscous and Tuna Stuffed Pepper

6 medium peppers	½ teaspoon salt
2 tablespoons oil	½ teaspoon cayenne pepper
1 large onion, sliced	1 7-ounce can tuna fish
2 cloves garlic, minced	3 tablespoons grated Parme-
½ cup mayonnaise	san cheese
1 teaspoon curry powder	½ cup couscous
1 teaspoon lemon juice	Paprika

Preheat oven to 350°.

Rinse and cut out stem ends from peppers, remove white fiber and seeds. Rinse the insides. Peppers can be stuffed, leaving just a hole at the stem ends, or they can be cut in half lengthwise.

Heat a large pot of salted water to the boiling point. Drop in peppers, and simmer for 5 minutes. Remove peppers and drain them.

Heat the oil in a skillet, add onion, and sauté until light brown. Add garlic and sauté 1 minute more. Add remaining ingredients except couscous and paprika and simmer for 10 minutes.

until light brown. Add garlic and sauté 1 minute more. Add couscous and simmer for 7 minutes.

Reserve ½ cup of tuna mixture for top of peppers.

Add couscous to remaining tuna mixture and stir well.

Place peppers in a large baking dish with enough water to cover bottom of dish. Spoon tuna mixture into peppers.

Divide the reserved tuna mixture over tops of the peppers. Sprinkle with paprika and bake for 15 minutes.

Makes 6 servings.

This dish can also be prepared with shrimp or other fish.

37.4 GRAMS PER SERVING

Kasha Stuffed Pepper

4 large peppers	1 teaspoon seasoned salt
2 tablespoons oil	½ teaspoon pepper
1 large onion, chopped	1 8-ounce can tomato sauce
2 cloves garlic	plus ½ can water
½ pound ground beef	½ cup kasha
1 teaspoon basil	Grated Parmesan cheese

Preheat oven to 350.°

Rinse and cut out stem ends from peppers, remove white fibers and seeds. Peppers can be stuffed leaving just a hole at the stem end, or they can be cut in half lengthwise. Heat a large pot of salted water to the boiling point, drop peppers in, and simmer for 5 minutes. Remove peppers and drain them.

Heat the oil in a skillet, add the chopped onion, and sauté until light brown. Add garlic and sauté 1 minute more. Add ground beef and sauté until brown. Add basil, seasoned salt, pepper, tomato sauce, and water.

Heat 1¼ cups salted water to the boiling point, add kasha, and simmer for 10 minutes.

Add kasha to ground beef mixture. Mix well.

Place peppers in baking dish with enough water to cover bottom of the dish. Spoon ground beef mixture in peppers. Sprinkle with Parmesan cheese. Bake for 15 minutes until tender.

Makes 4 servings.

19.2 GRAMS PER SERVING

Soya Couscous Dressing for Poultry

1¼ cups chicken broth
½ cup couscous
1 tablespoon butter
3 tablespoons oil
½ cup finely chopped onion
1 cup finely chopped celery
1 teaspoon sage
½ teaspoon marjoram

½ teaspoon thyme
1 teaspoon seasoned salt
½ cup slivered almonds (optional
1½ cups Hi-Protein Soya bread, cut into 1-inch cubes

Preheat oven to 350°.

Heat chicken broth to boiling, add couscous, turn to simmer, and cook for 7 minutes. Add butter and mix with a fork. Turn couscous into a colander, blanch with cold water, and break up any lumps with a fork.

In a skillet heat oil. Add onion and celery, sauté until golden brown; add sage, marjoram, thyme, salt, and almonds.

Add bread to onion mixture, add couscous, and mix well.

Place stuffing in a baking dish and bake for 20 minutes; or use to stuff poultry.

Makes 4 servings.

32.5 GRAMS PER SERVING

Scallops au Gratin

¾ cup cream
⅓ cup water
1½ cups diced Cheddar cheese
1 teaspoon mustard
1 teaspoon celery salt

½ teaspoon paprika
1 pound sea scallops
Juice of ½ lemon
½ cup Hi-Protein bread crumbs

Preheat oven to 350.°

Combine first 6 ingredients in a double boiler.

Simmer over low heat and stir constantly until smooth.

Place the scallops in a greased baking dish, and sprinkle with lemon juice.

Pour cheese sauce on scallops, and sprinkle with bread crumbs.

Bake for 30 minutes.

Makes 3 servings.

10.2 GRAMS PER SERVING

Grains

——◆——

Barley Pilaf

3 tablespoons butter
1 large onion, sliced
½ pound mushrooms, sliced

1 clove garlic, minced
1 cup pearl barley
3 cups chicken broth

Melt butter in a skillet. Sauté onion 2 minutes, add mushrooms, and sauté until golden; add garlic and sauté for 1 minute. Stir well.

Add barley and stir until golden brown. Add chicken broth, cover and simmer for 30 minutes or until broth is absorbed.

Makes 4 servings.

50.0 GRAMS PER SERVING

Bulgur Wheat and Barley Pilaf

3 tablespoons oil
2 medium carrots, chopped
1 large onion, sliced
1 cup sliced mushrooms
1 clove garlic, minced

½ cup bulgur wheat
½ cup barley
2¼ cups hot chicken broth
1 teaspoon basil
1 teaspoon seasoned salt

Heat oil in a skillet, sauté carrots, onion, and mushrooms until golden brown; add garlic at the last minute.

Add bulgur wheat and barley, stirring until well coated with oil.

Add chicken broth, basil, and salt. Stir again. Bring to a

boil. Cover and simmer for 25 to 30 minutes until broth is absorbed.

Makes 6 servings.

32.3 GRAMS PER SERVING

Millet with Mushrooms and Seeds

½ cup butter
1 large onion, chopped
½ pound mushrooms, sliced
1 clove garlic, minced
¾ cup millet
1 tablespoon marjoram

1 cup chicken broth
½ cup white wine
1 teaspoon salt
Dash pepper
½ cup pumpkin seeds

Heat butter in a skillet, sauté onion, mushrooms, and garlic until golden.

Add millet, and stir constantly until coated with butter.

Add marjoram, chicken broth, wine, salt, and pepper.

Cover and simmer for 30 minutes or until water is absorbed.

Stir in pumpkin seeds just before serving.

Makes 6 servings.

26.4 GRAMS PER SERVING

Sweet Baked Lentils

1 pound quick-cooking dried
    lentils
2 teaspoons salt
1 15-ounce can tomato sauce
½ cup honey

1 tablespoon prepared mus-
    tard
½ cup molasses
1 teaspoon onion powder
2 tablespoons minced onion

Preheat oven to 250°.

Place lentils, salt, and 4 cups water in large uncovered pot. Bring to a boil. Cover and simmer for 30 minutes.

Add remaining ingredients and pour into 2-quart casserole. Cover and bake for 2 hours.

Makes 8 servings.

57.1 GRAMS PER SERVING

Fried Rice

5 tablespoons peanut oil
4 eggs, lightly beaten
2 cups cooked, cold brown rice
10 slices bacon, sautéed and crumbled
½ cup chopped scallion
1 cup diced bamboo shoots
½ cup thinly sliced water chestnuts
½ cup diced green pepper
2 tablespoons soy sauce
2 teaspoons Worcestershire sauce

Heat 2 tablespoons oil in a large skillet. Add the eggs and scramble them. Push them to the side of skillet. Add remaining oil and rice; stir in with eggs.

Add remaining ingredients. Stir with a spatula, turning until heated thoroughly, about 10 minutes.

Makes 6 servings.

28.9 GRAMS PER SERVING

Vegetables

———◆———

Apple Cabbage

4 tablespoons safflower oil
1 medium red cabbage
8 medium red apples
½ teaspoon cinnamon
⅛ teaspoon ginger
⅛ teaspoon nutmeg

¼ cup cider vinegar
¾ cup honey
3 tablespoons unsweetened
   coconut marinated in 2
   tablespoons sherry

Wash and shred cabbage and sauté in oil in heavy skillet. Core apples and slice thin. Add to cabbage with spices, and stir well. Cook for 15 minutes, then remove from heat.

Add vinegar, honey, and marinated coconut (including marinade). Stir vigorously until apples dissolve.

Makes 8 servings.

37.5 GRAMS PER SERVING

Honey Baked Beans

2 cups dried lima beans
1 teaspoon salt
¼ pound bacon, diced
1 teaspoon salt
1 teaspoon dry mustard

1 teaspoon ground ginger
¾ cup honey
1 medium onion, diced
½ teaspoon ground cloves

Preheat oven to 350°.

Wash beans and drain. Soak in a large pan with water to cover.

Cook beans in same water, uncovered, until skins burst. Drain, and reserve liquid. Place beans in 2½-quart casserole with half of the bacon, remaining ingredients, and ½ cup bean liquid. Cover with the rest of the bacon.

Bake, covered, for 1½ hours. Remove cover for last ½ hour to brown top. Add more bean liquid while cooking if necessary.

Makes 8 servings.

29.7 GRAMS PER SERVING

Sweet and Sour Brown Beans

1 pound dried Idaho or
   Swedish brown beans
⅓ cup lemon juice
⅓ cup molasses

1 teaspoon salt
⅓ cup heavy cream
1 tablespoon parsley flakes

Boil 6 cups of water. Add washed beans and boil for 2 minutes. Cover, remove from heat, and let stand 1 hour. Return to heat, and simmer, covered, for 3 hours.

Add lemon juice, molasses, and salt. Stir in cream and blend well. Sprinkle with parsley. Serve.

Makes 8 servings.

17.5 GRAMS PER SERVING

Carrot Pudding

5 eggs, separated
¼ cup honey
2 tablespoons molasses
¾ cup grated carrots
½ cup chopped walnuts

¾ cup whole wheat flour,
   sifted
¼ cup soy flour, sifted
1 tablespoon wheat germ
1 teaspoon cinnamon
½ teaspoon ground cloves

Preheat oven to 350°.

Beat egg yolks, honey, and molasses until light and creamy. Add grated carrots, nuts, and flours. Beat egg whites until stiff peaks form. Fold into mix. Pour into 8-inch square greased baking pan, and sprinkle wheat germ, cinnamon, and cloves over top.

Bake for 45 minutes. If top becomes too brown, cover with foil to complete baking.

Makes 8 servings.

23.3 GRAMS PER SERVING

Carrot Ring

¾ cup oil
¼ cup molasses
¼ cup honey
1 teaspoon salt
1 tablespoon cold water
1 tablespoon lemon juice
1 tablespoon vanilla

3 eggs, separated
½ teaspoon baking powder
½ teaspoon baking soda
1 cup whole wheat flour
¼ cup soy flour
1 cup cooked carrots,
    mashed

Preheat oven to 350°.

Combine first 7 ingredients in large bowl. Mix well. Beat egg yolks until light and creamy and add them to the other ingredients.

Sift baking powder, baking soda, and flours. Mix well. Beat egg whites until peaks form, and fold in mixture. Bake in greased ring mold for 1 hour.

Makes 8 servings.

VARIATION: Pumpkin or butternut squash can be substituted for the carrots.

34.3 GRAMS PER SERVING

Green Beans au Gratin

3 tablespoons butter
1 medium onion, sliced
½ pound mushrooms, sliced
3 tablespoons soy flour
1 cup water
½ cup cream
1½ cups grated sharp cheese

1 teaspoon soy sauce
Salt and pepper to taste
2 cups cooked green beans
5-ounce can water chestnuts,
    drained and quartered
½ cup toasted slivered
    almonds

Preheat oven to 350°.

Melt butter in a skillet and sauté onion and mushrooms until golden.

Stir in soy flour and gradually add water and cream, stirring constantly until thickened. Add cheese, soy sauce, salt and pepper. Stir until cheese melts.

Add green beans and water chestnuts to cheese mixture. Place in an oiled baking dish. Sprinkle with almonds.

Bake for 30 minutes.

Makes 6 servings.

18 GRAMS PER SERVING

Hummus

2 cups cooked chick peas,
    drained
⅔ cup toasted ground
    sesame seeds
½ cup lemon juice
2 cloves garlic, minced

½ teaspoon curry powder
    (optional)
1 teaspoon salt
Dash cayenne
Fried pork rinds

Place all ingredients except cayenne and pork rinds in a blender and blend until smooth. Remove to a bowl, add cayenne.

Dip pork rinds into the hummus.
Makes 8 servings.

16.4 GRAMS PER SERVING

Lettuce and Peas

¼ cup butter
4 cups shredded lettuce
2 cups finely sliced onion
½ teaspoon salt
Dash pepper
½ teaspoon nutmeg

2 packages frozen peas,
    cooked and drained
½ teaspoon molasses
2 tablespoons toasted sesame
    seeds

Melt butter in heavy skillet. Add lettuce, onion, salt, pepper,
and nutmeg. Cook 5 minutes on low heat.

Add peas, molasses, and sesame seeds. Stir and cook until
peas are heated through.

Makes 8 servings.

20.3 GRAMS PER SERVING

Special Parsnips

1 pound parsnips
Boiling salted water
¼ cup butter

¼ cup honey
2 tablespoons toasted and
    chopped almonds

Trim and scrub parsnips. Cut in half crosswise, then cut each
half into two.

Boil, in water to cover, for 15 minutes. Drain. Add butter,
honey, and almonds. Cook over low heat, stirring gently, until glazed.

Makes 4 servings.

21.4 GRAMS PER SERVING

Pilaf with Chick Peas and Nuts

3 tablespoons butter
1 medium onion, finely
   chopped
1 clove garlic, minced
1 cup cooked chick peas,
   drained

1½ cups chicken broth
¾ cup brown rice
2 tablespoons parsley
½ cup chopped almonds or
   chopped pine nuts
Salt and pepper to taste

Heat butter in a large skillet and sauté onion till golden. Add garlic and sauté 1 minute longer.

Add remaining ingredients. Simmer for about 40 minutes until rice is done and water is absorbed. Allow to stand for 15 minutes before serving.

Makes 6 servings.

31.1 GRAMS PER SERVING

Special Squash

3 pounds yellow squash
2 cups water
1 teaspoon salt
¼ cup butter
2 cups diced onions
1 cup yogurt
½ teaspoon salt

¼ teaspoon pepper
¼ teaspoon ground thyme
¼ cup wheat germ
¾ cup fresh whole wheat
   bread crumbs
2 tablespoons melted butter
1 tablespoon paprika

Preheat oven to 350°.

Wash squash and cut into cubes. Place squash, water, and 1 teaspoon salt in covered saucepan. Bring to a boil, then reduce heat to simmer for 5 minutes. Drain well.

Melt ¼ cup butter in large skillet over medium heat. Add onion, stirring frequently until golden. Combine onion, squash, and yogurt. Add spices.

Pour into greased shallow casserole. Combine wheat germ, bread crumbs, melted butter, and paprika, and sprinkle over the top. Bake for 15 minutes to heat through, then place under broiler for 1 minute to brown crumbs.

Makes 8 servings.

30.5 GRAMS PER SERVING

Vegetable Omelet

4 tablespoons butter
¼ small eggplant, finely chopped
½ zucchini, finely chopped
¼ Bermuda onion, finely chopped

½ teaspoon garlic
4 eggs
1 tablespoon heavy cream
1 teaspoon seasoned salt
Freshly cracked black pepper

Melt 2 tablespoons butter in a skillet, add vegetables and garlic, and sauté for 6 minutes.

Melt remaining 2 tablespoons butter in an omelet pan. Beat eggs with cream, salt, and pepper. Beat vegetable mixture into eggs. Pour into omelet pan and tilt the pan to spread eggs to edges of pan.

Cook over a low flame until eggs begin to set. Loosen eggs from sides of pan with a spatula. Tilt pan again to allow uncooked egg mixture to spread to the sides.

Carefully fold the outer edges of the omelet into the center to resemble a flat cone. Slide omelet out of pan and serve.

Makes 2 servings.

This may be served as is, or with a sausage and tomato filling.

12 GRAMS PER SERVING

Wok Vegetables

4 tablespoons peanut oil
2 zucchini, sliced
½ small eggplant, diced
1 small onion, sliced
½ pound mushrooms, sliced

½ pound snow pea pods
2 tablespoons sesame seeds
2 tablespoons soy sauce
½ pound bean sprouts

Heat 2 tablespoons of oil in the wok. Add vegetables as listed. Cook zucchini, eggplant, and onions for 2 minutes. Add mushrooms and snow pea pods, and cook 2 minutes more. Add sesame seeds and soy sauce. Toss together well. Add bean sprouts. Cover the wok for 2 minutes more. Serve.
Makes 6 servings.

16.6 GRAMS PER SERVING

Zucchini Stuffed with Couscous

6 medium zucchini
3 tablespoons grated Parmesan cheese
4 tablespoons mayonnaise
6 slices lean prosciutto, diced

1 cup cooked couscous (page 154)
2 egg yolks
1 teaspoon seasoned salt
½ teaspoon pepper
1 teaspoon thyme
2 tablespoons olive oil

Preheat oven to 375°.

Bring a large pot of water to a boil, add zucchini, and boil for 5 minutes.

Drain zucchini and allow it to cool. Cut in half lengthwise, scoop out pulp, and save.

Mix together pulp from zucchini, 2 tablespoons Parmesan cheese and remaining ingredients, except olive oil.

Place zucchini halves in greased baking dish and fill each half with mixture.

Sprinkle with olive oil and remaining tablespoon Parmesan cheese.

Bake for 30 minutes.

Makes 12 servings.

16.93 GRAMS PER SERVING

Salads

———◆———

Avocado Cottage Cheese Mold

2 tablespoons gelatin
1 cup hot water
½ cup honey
1 cup cottage cheese
3 tablespoons mayonnaise
½ cup lemon juice

½ teaspoon salt
1 small avocado, cubed
1 cup honeydew melon
2 tablespoons chopped
    pimiento
Lettuce leaves

Dissolve gelatin in hot water. Add honey and stir.

Place cottage cheese, mayonnaise, lemon juice, and salt in a blender. Blend well.

Blend cheese mixture and gelatin and chill until partially set.

Carefully stir in remaining ingredients and place in a large mold. Chill until firm and serve on lettuce leaves.

Makes 6 servings.

23.9 GRAMS PER SERVING

Avocado and Egg Salad

1 avocado, cubed
1 small onion, chopped
1 teaspoon lemon juice
1 tablespoon lecithin gran-
    ules

Lettuce leaves
2 hard-boiled eggs, chopped
¼ cup Yogurt Dressing
    (page 235)

Combine avocado, onion, lemon juice, and lecithin.

Spoon on lettuce leaves. Sprinkle with chopped eggs and top with dressing.

Makes 4 servings.

9.4 GRAMS PER SERVING

Avocado Stuffed Tomato Salad

4 large, ripe tomatoes
1 avocado
2 teaspoons lemon juice
8 strips bacon
¼ pound fresh spinach, shredded

4 tablespoons Parmesan Caesar Dressing (page 111)

Scoop pulp out of tomato and reserve shells.

Peel avocado, dice, and sprinkle with lemon juice.

Fry bacon until crisp, drain, and crumble.

Combine avocado, bacon, and spinach. Add Caesar Dressing and mix well.

Fill tomato shells with the mixture.

Makes 4 lunch servings or 4 salad servings for dinner.

9.4 GRAMS PER SERVING

Summertime Bean Salad

2 cups cooked and drained kidney beans
2 cups cooked and drained garbanzo or green beans
1 medium onion, chopped
½ cup sliced celery
½ cup chopped cucumber
½ cup sliced mushrooms
¼ cup sliced ripe olives
⅓ cup olive oil

¼ cup wine vinegar
2 tablespoons mayonnaise
2 tablespoons tomato sauce
1 tablespoon honey
1 clove garlic, minced
1 teaspoon basil
2 teaspoons seasoned salt
¼ teaspoon Tabasco
2 hard-boiled eggs, sliced

Place beans in a large bowl. Add onion, celery, cucumber, mushrooms, and olives.

Prepare dressing with remaining ingredients, except eggs. Pour over beans and chill at least 1 hour.

Serve garnished with slices of egg.

Makes 10 servings.

8.4 GRAMS PER SERVING WITH GREEN BEANS
29.6 GRAMS PER SERVING WITH GARBANZO BEANS

Garbanzo Sprout Salad

1 cup cooked garbanzo beans	1 small zucchini, sliced
½ cup grated Parmesan cheese	½ cup grated Parmesan cheese
½ pound spinach	2 tablespoons lecithin granules
1 cup peas	½ cup Italian Dressing 1 or 2 (page 111)
6 scallions, sliced	
1 small green pepper, diced	

Combine all ingredients. Toss well.

Makes 4 servings.

48.6 GRAMS PER SERVING

Lentil Salad

1 cup dried lentils
1 medium onion, stuck with
    3 whole cloves
1 bay leaf
1 teaspoon salt
2 tablespoons safflower oil
1 tablespoon cider vinegar
2 tablespoons yogurt

½ teaspoon dried thyme
    leaves
½ clove garlic, crushed
¼ cup sliced onions
3 firm tomatoes, sliced
2 tablespoons chopped
    parsley

Combine lentils, onion, bay leaf, and salt with 3 cups water. Bring to a boil and simmer until tender (about 40 minutes). Drain, and discard onion and bay leaf.

Mix together oil, vinegar, yogurt, thyme, garlic, and sliced onion. Add lentils, and toss gently to combine.

Place in serving dish, and garnish with sliced tomatoes and parsley.

Makes 6 servings.

25.3 GRAMS PER SERVING

Peanut and Carrot Salad

1 cup peanut butter
2 tablespoons honey
4 cups cooked brown rice
2 cups shredded carrots

1 cup unsweetened coconut
1 tablespoon safflower oil
½ teaspoon salt
Lettuce leaves

Stir together peanut butter and honey. Add remaining ingredients except lettuce leaves.

Chill well. Serve on bed of lettuce.

Makes 8 servings.

45.8 GRAMS PER SERVING

Hot Peas and Olive Salad

2 tablespoons butter
1 tablespoon chopped onion
1 tablespoon chopped celery
1 tablespoon chopped green
    pepper
¼ teaspoon oregano
1 packet sugar substitute

Dash cayenne pepper
3 tablespoons finely chopped
    pimiento
¼ cup chopped black olives
1 package frozen peas,
    cooked, or fresh peas,
    steamed

Melt the butter in a skillet and sauté the onion until it softens. Add celery and green pepper and sauté until golden. Add remaining ingredients except peas. Stir together until blended.

Remove from heat and refrigerate for 1 hour. Add peas and reheat.

Makes 4 servings.

19.6 GRAMS PER SERVING

Curried Tuna Rice Salad

3 cups chicken broth
1¼ cups brown rice
2 tablespoons soy grits
2 teaspoons curry powder
1 small onion, minced
2 6½- or 7-ounce cans tuna,
    drained
½ cup diced celery

¼ cup diced green pepper
4 scallions, sliced
½ cup cream
½ cup yogurt
Lettuce leaves
1 cup salted peanuts
½ cup coconut

This salad should be prepared several hours in advance.

Bring chicken broth to a boil. Add rice, soy grits, curry powder, and onion. Cover and simmer for 45 minutes. Chill.

Place tuna chunks, celery, green pepper, and scallions in a large bowl. Chill.

About 2 hours before serving, whip cream until stiff and fold in yogurt. Gently stir into tuna mixture with chilled rice. Cover and chill.

To serve, spoon on lettuce leaves and sprinkle with peanuts and coconut.

Makes 8 servings.

22.6 GRAMS PER SERVING

Sauces

Barbecue Spread

½ pound butter
1 teaspoon dry mustard
1 teaspoon salt
1 teaspoon paprika
1 clove garlic, mashed
2 tablespoons honey
2 tablespoons lemon juice

¼ cup chopped onion
2 tablespoons Worcestershire
sauce
1 tablespoon tomato sauce
2 drops Tabasco
2 tablespoons wine vinegar

Soften butter. Blend in mustard, salt, and paprika. Beat in
remaining ingredients. Store in refrigerator.
Makes 1½ cups.

TOTAL GRAMS 33.2

Sweet Barbecue Sauce

2 tablespoons dry mustard
¼ cup tomato sauce
½ cup honey

½ cup orange juice
1 teaspoon lemon juice

Combine all ingredients. Allow them to blend by storing for
1 hour before using.
Makes 1 cup (16 tablespoons).

TOTAL GRAMS 110.6
6.9 PER TABLESPOON

Spanish Sausage Sauce for Beans

½ pound hot Italian sausage	1 tablespoon rum
2 tablespoons butter	⅛ teaspoon cinnamon
1 medium onion, sliced	Salt and pepper to taste
2 cloves garlic, minced	¼ cup olive oil
½ cup tomatoes	2 tablespoons wheat germ
1 cup water	(optional)
¼ cup pine nuts	6 cups cooked white kidney beans

Sauté sausage in an ungreased skillet. Prick with a fork and simmer until brown. Pour off the oil from sausages. Cool and remove skin.

Melt butter in medium skillet. Sauté onion and garlic to light brown. Add tomatoes, water, pine nuts, rum, cinnamon, salt, pepper, and sausage. Simmer 15 minutes. Add olive oil and wheat germ.

Place in blender and blend to a fine puree.

Serve the beans in a bowl and spoon sauce on top.

Makes 8 servings.

40.1 GRAMS PER SERVING WITH KIDNEY BEANS

Cranberry Sauce

2½ cups fresh cranberries	2 tablespoons Cranberry or Orange liqueur
1½ cups water	1 tablespoon diet orange syrup
1 package diet lemon or orange gelatin	Pinch salt
8 packets sugar substitute	

Cook cranberries in water over low heat until they pop open. Drain and press through sieve, and add boiling water until there are 1½ cups liquid.

Dissolve gelatin, sugar substitute, and flavorings in hot liquid.

Chill until firm. Slice to serve.

Makes 6 servings.

11.2 GRAMS PER SERVING

Strawberry and Raspberry Sauce

½ cup fresh strawberries
½ cup fresh raspberries
½ bottle diet strawberry soda
1½ teaspoons arrowroot powder
2 teaspoons cold water

1 teaspoon Cointreau
1 teaspoon Strawberry liqueur
2 packets sugar substitute
1 can mandarin oranges (packed in water), drained

Heat strawberries and raspberries in diet soda until softened. Remove from heat. Dissolve arrowroot powder in water. Stir into berry mixture and heat until thickened. Add liqueurs, sugar substitute, and oranges. Serve.

Makes 4 servings.

11.1 GRAMS PER SERVING

Breads

———————

Whole Wheat Bread

2 tablespoons yeast
3½ cups warm stock*
2 eggs
½ cup honey
½ cup oil
3 tablespoons lecithin granules

1 cup wheat germ
1 cup soya flour
1 cup bran
1 cup ground sesame seeds
2 teaspoons salt
9–10 cups whole wheat flour

Preheat oven to 350°.

Dissolve yeast in warm stock in a large bowl. (*It is very important that the temperature is not too cold or hot: it should be body temperature.) Let it set for 5 minutes, then stir until dissolved.

Add eggs, honey or molasses, and oil. Stir well.

Add remaining ingredients except whole wheat flour. Beat well.

Gradually add whole wheat flour. When dough is stiff enough to knead, place on a floured breadboard and knead, adding more flour until the dough is smooth and elastic. If the dough does not seem smooth enough, let it rest for 15 minutes covered. Knead again.

Place the dough back in the large bowl, brush the top with oil, cover with a damp towel. Turn oven on to its lowest point for 2 minutes, turn off, and place bowl in warm oven. Let it rise for 4 to 5 hours, until it doubles in size. Knead again for 5 minutes, shape into 4 loaves, and place them in 4 oiled loaf pans. Place them back in the warm oven to rise again for 1 or more hours until doubled in size again. Bake loaves 30 to 40 minutes until they are nicely brown and sound hollow when tapped on top.

Makes 24 thin slices per loaf.

13.6 GRAMS PER SLICE

Sesame Seed Breadsticks

Prepare Whole Wheat Bread recipe (page 177)
Preheat oven to 350°.
Knead dough before second rising.
For each breadstick, pinch off a piece of the dough the size of a large walnut. Roll between hands or on a breadboard to make a roll 8–10 inches long.
Brush with oil and roll in sesame seeds. Let rise until double in bulk. Bake for 30 minutes.
Makes 20 breadsticks.

13 GRAMS PER BREADSTICK

Zucchini Bread

½ cup peanut oil
¾ cup honey
¼ cup molasses
3 cups grated zucchini
½ cup chopped walnuts
1 teaspoon salt
⅓ cup yogurt
1 teaspoon cinnamon

1 teaspoon ground cloves
2 eggs
1 tablespoon baking powder
1½ cups whole wheat flour
¼ cup soya flour
¼ cup wheat germ
¼ cup ground nut meal

Preheat oven to 350°.
Combine oil, honey, molasses, zucchini, walnuts, salt, yogurt, cinnamon, cloves, and eggs. Mix well.
Stir in remaining ingredients. Spoon mixture into a well-greased 9 × 5-inch loaf pan. Bake 1 hour or until knife inserted in middle comes out clean.
Makes 12 servings.

TOTAL GRAMS 467.7
39.0 GRAMS PER SERVING

Desserts

◆

Cream Puffs

2 cups water
¼ cup butter
1 cup soya flour
1 packet sugar substitute
½ teaspoon Ouzo

½ teaspoon orange extract
2 eggs
1 package diet vanilla pudding mix
2 tablespoons heavy cream

Preheat oven to 400°.

Boil 1 cup water. Add cut-up butter and dissolve. Add soya flour, sugar substitute, Ouzo, and orange extract. Simmer for 2 minutes. Remove from heat. Add eggs and mix well. Place dough in waxed paper and refrigerate for 1 hour.

Place batter into greased mini muffin tins. Bake for 30 minutes until golden brown. Remove to rack. Cool slightly. *Invert* muffins, scoop out each center, and reserve for cookie crumbs. Allow to cool thoroughly.

Meanwhile, prepare vanilla pudding using heavy cream and 1 cup water.

Add pudding by teaspoons to puff centers.

Makes 8 cream puffs.

10.2 GRAMS PER CREAM PUFF

Apple Nut Pinwheels

¾ cup honey
¼ cup lemon juice
¼ cup water
1½ cups whole wheat flour
1 teaspoon salt
3 teaspoons baking powder
½ cup butter
½ cup rolled oats

½ cup heavy cream
½ cup butter, melted
2 tablespoons molasses
1 tablespoon cinnamon
1 teaspoon nutmeg
1½ cups diced unpeeled
    apple
1 cup chopped nuts

Preheat oven to 400°.

Mix honey, lemon juice, and water. Bring to a boil in small pot; remove from heat and cool.

Mix flour, salt, and baking powder. Cut in ½ cup butter until mixture resembles coarse crumbs. Add oats and cream, and mix lightly until dough clears the bowl.

Roll out to form a 13×9-inch rectangle. Brush with melted butter. Mix 2 tablespoons melted butter, molasses, cinnamon, nutmeg, apples, and nuts. Sprinkle on dough and roll up, sealing edges. Cut in 1½-inch slices and arrange in 13×9-inch pan.

Pour honey syrup over top and bake for 20 minutes.
Makes 8 servings.

57.9 GRAMS PER SERVING

Pumpkin Nut Cookies

¼ cup butter
½ cup honey
1 egg, beaten
½ cup canned pumpkin
¾ cup whole wheat flour,
    sifted
¼ cup soy flour, sifted

2 teaspoons baking powder
½ teaspoon salt
1 teaspoon cinnamon
½ teaspoon nutmeg
¼ teaspoon ground cloves
⅛ teaspoon ground ginger
½ cup chopped walnuts

Preheat oven to 350°.

Cream butter and add honey, egg, and pumpkin. Mix well.

Sift flours, baking powder, salt, and spices together. Stir into pumpkin mixture, adding nuts.

Drop by teaspoonfuls onto greased cookie sheet. Bake for 15 minutes.

Makes 2 dozen cookies.

11.1 GRAMS PER COOKIE

Tahini Cookies

6 tablespoons tahini (sesame seed butter)
¼ cup honey
¼ cup molasses

½ cup chopped walnuts
1½ cups instant oatmeal
½ teaspoon cinnamon
¼ teaspoon nutmeg

Preheat oven to 350°.

Stir tahini, honey, and molasses together. Add nuts and stir well. Add oatmeal, cinnamon, and nutmeg, and blend well.

Drop by teaspoonfuls onto greased cookie sheet. Bake for 10 minutes.

Makes 2 dozen cookies.

25.7 GRAMS PER COOKIE

Nut Muffins

¼ cup butter
1 cup soya flour
1 tablespoon wheat germ
2 teaspoons baking powder

1 packet sugar substitute
2 eggs, beaten
1 teaspoon vanilla
½ cup chopped nuts

Preheat oven to 375°.

Boil ½ cup water in saucepan. Add cut-up pieces of butter to boiling water. Stir to dissolve. Add flour, wheat germ, baking powder, and sugar substitute. Mix well and remove from heat. Add eggs, vanilla, and nuts. Mix well.

Drop by spoonfuls on a greased cookie sheet, spacing 1½ inches apart. Bake for 12 to 15 minutes.

Makes 8 muffins.

4.4 GRAMS PER MUFFIN

Orange Bran Muffins

4 eggs, separated	1 cup ground almonds
2 packets sugar substitute	2 tablespoons bran
1 tablespoon fructose	1 teaspoon baking powder
4 tablespoons fresh orange juice	1 tablespoon soya flour
1 teaspoon orange extract	1 tablespoon wheat germ

Preheat oven to 375°.

Whisk egg yolks, sugar substitute, fructose, orange juice, and orange extract. Add almonds, bran, baking powder, soya flour, and wheat germ.

Beat whites to stiff peaks, fold into yolk mixture. Pour into 12 greased muffin tins. Bake for 40 minutes.

Makes 12 muffins.

8.0 GRAMS PER SERVING

Orange Pecan Muffins

1½ cups whole wheat flour	½ cup melted butter
½ cup soy flour	1 cup sour cream
2 teaspoons baking powder	1 tablespoon grated orange rind
1 teaspoon baking soda	1 cup chopped pecans
1 teaspoon salt	2 teaspoons vanilla
2 eggs	
½ cup honey	

Preheat oven to 375°.

Oil muffin tins.

Combine first 5 ingredients in a mixing bowl and stir.

In a separate bowl, beat eggs lightly, add honey, butter, sour cream, and orange rind. Add flour mixture, pecans, and vanilla.

Fill muffin tins ⅔ full. Bake 20 to 25 minutes.

Makes 24 muffins.

12.8 GRAMS PER SERVING

Orange Health Loaf

3 eggs, separated
1 packet sugar substitute
1 tablespoon fructose
3 tablespoons fresh orange juice

1 teaspoon vanilla extract
1 cup ground almonds
1 teaspoon baking powder
2 tablespoons soya flour

Preheat oven to 375°.

Whisk egg yolks, sugar substitute, fructose, orange juice, and vanilla. Add almonds, baking powder, and soya flour.

Beat whites to stiff peaks; fold into yolk mixture. Pour into greased 9×5×3-inch loaf pan.

Bake for 40 minutes.

Makes 8 servings.

TOTAL GRAMS 49
6.1 GRAMS PER SERVING

Note: Fructose may be omitted. When cake is removed from oven, spread 2 tablespoons Orange liqueur on top.

TOTAL GRAMS 55.0
6.9 GRAMS PER SERVING

Special Brownies

½ cup butter
1 cup honey
1 egg
1½ cups whole wheat flour, sifted
¼ cup soy flour, sifted

2 tablespoons wheat germ
2 teaspoons baking powder, sifted
½ teaspoon salt
1½ cups grated carrots
½ cup chopped walnuts

Preheat oven to 350°.

Melt butter in saucepan. Add honey and stir well. Remove from heat and beat in egg. Add all dry ingredients slowly and beat well. Lightly mix in carrots and nuts.

Pour batter into 13×9×2-inch greased pan. Bake for 30 minutes. Cool and cut into squares.

Makes 2 dozen brownies.

16.2 GRAMS PER SERVING

Poppy Seed Cake

½ pound butter
1 cup honey
¼ cup molasses
4 egg yolks, well beaten
2 tablespoons poppy seeds
1 teaspoon baking soda

1 cup yogurt
1¾ cups whole wheat pastry flour, sifted
¼ cup soy flour, sifted
1 teaspoon vanilla
4 egg whites, stiffly beaten

Preheat oven to 350°.

Cream butter. Add honey and molasses and blend well. Mix together the egg yolks and poppy seeds, and add to butter mixture, stirring thoroughly.

Add soda to yogurt, and add alternately with the flours, beating well after each addition.

Add vanilla. Beat thoroughly.

Fold egg whites into batter.

Bake in 10-inch ungreased tube pan for 1 hour, or until cake tester comes out clean.

Makes 10 servings.

36.4 GRAMS PER SERVING

Rum Couscous Pudding

½ cup couscous
½ cup cream
Dash salt
2 tablespoons butter
2 eggs

1 teaspoon rum extract
1 teaspoon lemon juice
1 teaspoon grated lemon
  rind

Preheat oven to 350°.

Heat 1¼ cups of water to boiling. Add couscous and simmer 7 minutes.

Heat cream and ½ cup water, do not boil. Add salt, butter, eggs, rum extract, lemon juice, lemon rind, and couscous. Mix well.

Pour mixture into an oiled baking dish. Bake about 1 hour or until center is set.

Makes 4 servings.

23.7 GRAMS PER SERVING

Baked Brown Rice Pudding

½ cup brown rice
¾ cup cream
2 eggs
4 tablespoons honey
1 teaspoon vanilla

1 teaspoon nutmeg
1 teaspoon cinnamon
½ cup pumpkin seeds or
  walnuts

Preheat oven to 350°.

Heat 1¼ cups water to boiling, add rice, and simmer 30 minutes.

Heat cream and 1½ cups water together in a pot (do not boil).

Meanwhile, combine eggs, honey, and vanilla. Add hot cream and water to egg mixture. Add rice and seeds or nuts. Mix well. Pour into an oiled baking dish; sprinkle nutmeg and cinnamon on top.

Bake about 1 hour or until center is set.

Makes 6 servings.

15.8 GRAMS PER SERVING

Caramel Cream

1 cup cream
1 cup water
4 tablespoons couscous
3 tablespoons honey

1 tablespoon melted butter
1 teaspoon vanilla
½ teaspoon salt

Preheat oven to 225°.

Combine all ingredients in a baking dish. Blend well.

Bake 3 hours, stirring every half hour until couscous is dissolved. Serve with a topping of whipped cream or nuts.

Makes 4½ cups.

19.9 GRAMS PER SERVING

Halvah

½ cup finely ground unsweetened coconut
½ cup sunflower seed meal
½ cup natural wheat germ

¼ cup tahini (ground sesame seed)
¼ cup honey
¼ cup finely chopped nuts

Mix all ingredients together and shape into thin rectangle. Wrap in waxed paper and refrigerate until chilled. Cut into square chunks to serve.

Makes 10 servings.

22.5 GRAMS PER SERVING

Strawberry Mold

1 8-ounce package cream cheese, softened
¼ cup sour cream
4 packets sugar substitute
1 tablespoon lemon juice
½ teaspoon salt

1 cup sliced strawberries
½ cup pine nuts
½ cup chopped walnuts
1 tablespoon lecithin granules (optional)
1 cup whipped cream

Combine cream cheese, sour cream, sugar substitute, lemon juice, and salt. Beat until light and fluffy.

Fold in strawberries, nuts, and lecithin. Fold in cream. Place in a mold and chill until firm. Unmold.

Makes 6 servings.

10.7 GRAMS PER SERVING

Josie's Trifle

1 package diet orange gelatin
1 package diet strawberry gelatin
1 package diet vanilla pudding mix
½ Light Sponge Cake (page 121)

2 tablespoons Port wine
2 tablespoons brandy
¼ cup unsweetened coconut
1 cup sliced strawberries
1 cup cream
½ cup chopped walnuts

Dissolve orange gelatin in 1½ cups of boiling water and refrigerate until slightly firm.

Dissolve strawberry gelatin in 1½ cups boiling water and refrigerate until slightly firm.

Make pudding mix according to directions and refrigerate until slightly firm.

Cut sponge cake into 2×1-inch rectangles and place in a large glass bowl. Sprinkle with Port wine and brandy. Spoon orange gelatin over sponge cake. Sprinkle coconut over gelatin. Spoon vanilla pudding over coconut. Spoon strawberry gelatin over pudding. Add strawberries to the bowl.

Whip cream until thick and spoon over the strawberries. Sprinkle walnuts over the cream.

Refrigerate trifle for 2 hours, or until ready to serve.

Makes 8 servings.

10.6 GRAMS PER SERVING

Beverages

Banana Apple Whip

2 cups Apple tea (available in specialty and health food stores)
3 tablespoons cream
1 banana
1 packet sugar substitute
1 teaspoon brewer's yeast

Place all ingredients in blender. Blend well.
Makes 2 servings.

6.7 GRAMS PER SERVING

Pumpkin Punch

½ cup honey
1 teaspoon cinnamon
½ teaspoon nutmeg
¼ teaspoon ground cloves
½ cup cream
2 eggs
1 can pumpkin
1 cup club soda
1 cup grapefruit juice

Blend all ingredients except club soda and grapefruit juice.
To serve, combine with soda and juice in a punchbowl.
Makes 12 servings.

11.6 GRAMS PER SERVING

Sweet Lemonade with Lecithin

1 cup water
¼ cup lemon juice
¼ cup honey
2 egg whites
1 teaspoon vanilla

½ teaspoon orange extract
Dash of salt
8 ice cubes
2 teaspoons lecithin

Place all ingredients except ice cubes and lecithin in a blender. Blend until thick.

Add 1 ice cube at a time and blend until frothy.

Remove from blender and stir in lecithin. Pour into 4 glasses. Stir again and serve immediately.

Makes 4 servings.

18.8 GRAMS PER SERVING

DIET 3

MENU PLAN
FOR DIET 3

DAY ONE

Breakfast:

Bacon
    Two slices French Toast using
      Hi-Protein Soya Bread

Lunch:

Salad Niçoise
    Coffee or tea

Dinner:

Onion Soup
    Chicken Paprika
      Winter Squash
        Cherry D-Zerta

Snack:

Two Frozen Peanut Candies

DAY TWO

Breakfast:

  Blueberry jam omelet
    Coffee

Lunch:

  Creamy Tomato Avocado Soup
    Summer Salad 1
      Coffee or tea

Dinner:

  Sole with Nut and Seed Sauce
    Pungent Cabbage
      Coffee or tea

Snack:

  One piece Chocolate Fudge

DAY THREE

Breakfast:

Mocha Bran Shake

Lunch:

Green Salad
Pumpkin Soup
Coffee or tea

Dinner:

Armenian Stew
Cold Green Bean Salad with Nuts
Coffee or tea

Snack:

Sweet Melon

DAY FOUR

Breakfast:

Nut-Bran Shake
Scrambled eggs
Coffee or tea

Lunch:

Crisp Chinese Salad
Strawberry Cheese Pudding

Dinner:

Crabmeat with Cheese
Carrots and Herbs

Snack:

Two pieces Oatmeal-Carob Nut Candy

DAY FIVE

Breakfast:

> Two poached eggs
>> Two slices Hi-Protein Soya Bread
>>> Coffee

Lunch:

> Turkey Salad
>> Acapulco Chicken Soup
>>> Coffee or tea

Dinner:

> Hot Borscht
>> Eggplant Stew
>>> Coffee or tea

Snack:

> Two Popcorn Balls

DAY SIX

Breakfast:

Ham and cheese omelet
Coffee

Lunch:

Healthy Cottage Cheese Salad
Coffee or tea

Dinner:

Curried Chicken Avocado
Cauliflower with Nuts and Seeds
Coffee or tea

Snack:

Two pieces Peanut Butter Sesame Seed Candy

DAY SEVEN

Breakfast:

Bacon
  Cheese omelet
    Coffee

Lunch:

Bean Sprout Salad
  Uncooked Cottage Cheese Pudding
    Coffee or tea

Dinner:

Cream of Asparagus Soup with Nuts
  Hearty Seafood Salad
    Coffee or tea

Snack:

2 pieces Carob Sesame Seed Candy

RECIPES
FOR DIET 3

———◆———

Appetizers

———◆———

Curry Dip

4 small garlic cloves
2 teaspoons curry powder
1 cup sour cream

2 teaspoons chopped parsley
1 teaspoon horseradish
1 teaspoon seasoned salt

Crush the garlic cloves and combine with the remaining ingredients. Mix thoroughly and chill.

TOTAL GRAMS 19.1

Health-Stuffed Celery

8 stalks celery
1 medium avocado
2 green peppers, minced

½ cup ground sunflower seeds
1 tablespoon lecithin granules (optional)

Wash and dry celery. Cut in half.

Mash avocado with a fork, add minced green pepper, sunflower seeds, and lecithin. Mix well. Spoon mixture into celery stalks. Cut stalks in thirds.

Makes 12 servings.

8.1 GRAMS PER SERVING

Fried Mozzarella Cheese

½ pound Mozzarella cheese
2 eggs, beaten
¼ teaspoon salt

1 cup Hi-Protein bread
    crumbs
Olive oil for frying

Cut Mozzarella into 4-inch squares. Dip cheese squares in eggs and salt, then in bread crumbs, then back in eggs and bread crumbs again.

Heat olive oil in a skillet. Fry cheese cubes until golden brown. Serve immediately.

Makes 4 servings.

9.2 GRAMS PER SERVING

Oysters Rockefeller

24 oysters on the half shell
1 cup butter
⅓ cup finely chopped
    parsley
¼ cup finely chopped celery
¼ cup finely chopped
    shallots or scallions
½ clove garlic, minced

2 cups chopped watercress
⅓ cup chopped fennel
⅓ cup fine, soft Hi-Protein
    bread crumbs
¼ cup Pernod
Salt and freshly ground pep-
    per to taste

Preheat oven to 450°.

Fill 4 10-inch pie plates with rock salt and arrange 6 oysters on each.

Heat the butter in a skillet and add the parsley, celery, shallots and garlic. Cook 3 minutes. Add the watercress and fennel and cook about 1 minute more—until the watercress wilts.

Pour the cooked mixture into a blender and add bread crumbs, and Pernod. Blend until the sauce is thoroughly pureed, about 1 minute. Add salt and pepper to taste.

Place 1 tablespoon of the sauce on each oyster and spread to the rim of the shell.

Bake about 4 minutes—just until sauce bubbles.

Makes 4 servings.

10.8 GRAMS PER SERVING

Crabmeat with Cheese

¾ cup minced onion
¼ cup peanut oil
2 tablespoons curry powder
1 pound crabmeat, flaked and picked over
2 tablespoons minced parsley
¼ teaspoon crushed red pepper

2 tablespoons lemon juice
½ teaspoon seasoned salt
½ teaspoon black pepper
¼ teaspoon oregano
½ cup grated Parmesan cheese
2 tablespoons butter
1 lemon, cut into wedges

Sauté the onion in peanut oil until it is soft. Add the curry powder and cook, stirring constantly, for 1 minute.

Stir in the crabmeat, parsley, and red pepper, and sauté for 2 minutes. Add the lemon juice, salt, pepper, and oregano. Sauté for 1 minute more.

Divide the crabmeat mixture among 4 buttered scallop shells, sprinkle each serving with Parmesan cheese, and dot the tops with butter. Put the shells under the broiler for 2 to 3 minutes, or until the cheese is golden. Serve the shells with wedges of lemon.

Makes 4 servings.

8.7 GRAMS PER SERVING

Soups

Acapulco Chicken Soup

6 cups beef stock or bouillon
1 small onion, minced
½ cup millet or couscous
2 chicken breasts, cooked
    and cut into large strips

1 canned whole green chili
    pepper
1 tablespoon chopped parsley
1 small avocado, cut into
    strips

Heat the stock. Add remaining ingredients except avocado strips.

Cover and simmer for 7 minutes. Remove chili pepper and discard.

Garnish with avocado strips and serve.

Makes 4 servings.

15.5 GRAMS PER SERVING

Apple Curry Soup

1 tablespoon butter
½ cup chopped onion
½ cup chopped celery
12 ounces apple juice
2 cups chicken bouillon or
    broth
½ teaspoon curry powder

1 teaspoon lemon juice
1 teaspoon honey
Apple slivers from 1 un-
    peeled apple
⅓ cup heavy cream,
    whipped

Melt butter in a saucepan over low heat. Add onion and celery, and sauté until golden brown. Add the juices, and cook, stirring, about 10 minutes.

Add bouillon, curry powder, lemon juice, and honey. Cook 2 minutes longer. Strain. Pour soup into individual bowls over apple slivers. Place a dollop of whipped cream in center of each bowl.

Makes 8 servings.

9.5 GRAMS PER SERVING

Cream of Asparagus Soup with Nuts

2 pounds fresh asparagus	6 cups chicken broth
3 tablespoons butter	¼ cup dry sherry
1 cup whole blanched almonds	Salt and pepper to taste
	½ cup heavy cream
1 medium onion, chopped	2 tablespoons lecithin granules (optional)
1 cup chopped celery	
1 cup diced ham	

Wash and cut tips from asparagus. Cover and simmer tips in a small amount of water until tender.

Heat butter in a large pot and sauté almonds, onion, celery, and ham until almonds are light brown, and onion and celery are soft.

Combine almond mixture with chopped asparagus stalks (without tips) in a blender. Add a little chicken broth and blend to a smooth paste.

Heat remaining chicken broth in a large pot, add sherry, salt, pepper, and mixture from the blender. Stir well, cover, and simmer for 15 minutes.

Turn heat off and add cream, asparagus tips, and lecithin. Reheat, but do not boil.

Makes 6 servings.

16.4 GRAMS PER SERVING

Hot Borscht

1 pound lean beef, cubed
1½ quarts water
1 tablespoon salt
1½ cups shredded raw beets
¾ cup shredded carrots
¾ cup shredded white
    turnips
1 medium onion, chopped

2 tablespoons tomato puree
2 tablespoons butter
2 tablespoons lemon juice
1 teaspoon honey
½ small cabbage, shredded
Black pepper to taste
3 bay leaves
½ cup sour cream

Simmer beef in salted water about 1½ hours. Sauté the beets, carrots, turnips, onion, and tomato puree in butter with lemon juice and honey, covered, for 15 minutes. Stir frequently. Add shredded cabbage to vegetables and sauté 10 minutes longer.

Combine cooked beef, vegetables, pepper to taste, and bay leaves in meat pan. Cook, covered, for a few minutes to combine flavors. Remove bay leaves and add sour cream.

Makes 10 servings.

7.4 GRAMS PER SERVING

Creamy Cauliflower Soup

6 cups chicken broth
3 medium leeks, thinly sliced
3 medium carrots, pared and
    sliced thin
2 large onions, peeled and
    sliced
1 teaspoon ground cloves
1 teaspoon dried marjoram
    leaves
¼ teaspoon ground celery
    seed

¼ teaspoon white pepper
½ teaspoon ground nutmeg
1 teaspoon salt
2-pound head cauliflower or
    2 packages frozen
½ cup heavy cream
2 egg yolks
1 tablespoon arrowroot flour
8 ounces grated Swiss cheese

Heat broth. Add spices and vegetables (except cauliflower) and bring to a boil. Reduce heat and simmer, covered, 15 minutes.

Meanwhile, wash and separate cauliflower into flowerets. Add them to the soup, bring it back to a boil, then reduce heat to simmer, and cook uncovered for 30 minutes.

In a small bowl, combine cream, egg yolks, and arrowroot. Whisk until smooth. Stir in a little of the hot soup and whisk well. Pour into soup pot and bring to a boil, stirring.

Put in ovenproof casserole with grated cheese sprinkled on top. Place under broiler for 2-3 minutes to melt cheese.

Makes 8 servings.

14.7 GRAMS PER SERVING

Onion Soup

6 **small onions, sliced thin**	**Salt and pepper to taste**
2 **tablespoons butter**	6 **slices Hi-Protein Soya**
1 **teaspoon arrowroot flour**	**Bread (page 115),**
6 **cups beef stock or**	**toasted**
consommé	3 **tablespoons grated Swiss**
½ **cup dry white wine**	**cheese**

Lightly brown the onions in butter. Sprinkle with flour, and add the consommé, wine, and salt and pepper to taste. Simmer for 15 minutes.

Place toast in the bottom of an ovenproof soup tureen. Pour the soup over the toast, sprinkle with grated cheese, and put the tureen under the broiler to melt the cheese. (May also be prepared in individual soup crocks.)

Makes 6 servings.

12.3 GRAMS PER SERVING

Pumpkin Soup

½ cup chopped onion
2 tablespoons butter
2 cups chicken broth
1 teaspoon pumpkin pie
    spice
½ teaspoon ground cloves
¼ teaspoon salt
Pinch pepper

2 cups yogurt
1 cup canned solid-pack
    pumpkin
½ cup chopped fresh
    tomatoes, peeled and
    drained
2 tablespoons chopped chives

Sauté chopped onion in butter. Add 1 cup of chicken broth and all the spices. Bring to boil and simmer, covered, 10 minutes. Add yogurt and pumpkin, and blend. Add remaining cup of chicken broth. Stir well.

Heat gently until very hot, but do not boil. Garnish with tomatoes and chives.

Makes 6 servings.

9.1 GRAMS PER SERVING

Creamy Tomato Avocado Soup

2½ cups Tomato Soup,
    heated (page 211)
1 tomato, peeled and sliced
Dash pepper

3-ounce package cream
    cheese, softened
1 teaspoon chopped chives
Small ripe avocado, sliced
    thin

Place heated tomato soup in a saucepan with the tomato slices and simmer 5 minutes. Add pepper.

Mix cream cheese and chives and beat until fluffy. Pour hot soup into individual bowls. Place a heaping tablespoon of cheese in the center and garnish with avocado slices. Serve immediately.

Makes 4 servings.

9.7 GRAMS PER SERVING

Red Harvest Soup

2 tablespoons butter
3 carrots, diced
1½ cups chopped onion
1 stalk celery with leaves, diced
1 lamb chop, or beef scraps and bones
6 cups water
1 teaspoon thyme
3 leeks, diced
½ head cauliflower, cut into flowerets

1 zucchini, diced
1 grean pepper, diced
1 red pepper, diced
1 small eggplant, peeled and diced
2½ cups tomato juice
2 teaspoons Capsicum tea
1 teaspoon oregano
1 teaspoon sweet basil
Salt to taste

Sauté carrots, 1 cup diced onion, and celery in butter for 3-5 minutes until soft. Add meat, bones, water, and thyme. Simmer for 1 hour. Strain and reserve stock.

To 4 cups stock add remaining ingredients. Bring to a boil and simmer covered for 45 minutes.

Makes 8 servings.

17.3 GRAMS PER SERVING

Greek Egg and Lemon Soup

1 chicken, quartered
½ cup chopped celery
2 bouillon cubes
2 quarts water

Salt and pepper to taste
½ cup brown rice
6 eggs
Juice of 4 lemons

Place chicken, celery, bouillon cubes, water, salt, and pepper into a pot. Cover and boil for 45 minutes. Add rice and cook another 20 minutes until rice is tender. Remove from heat.

Skin, bone, and cut chicken into small pieces and set aside.

Beat eggs until light and frothy. Slowly beat in lemon juice and 2 cups broth. Mix well.

Add the egg and lemon mixture, chicken, and the rest of broth and rice. Place on a *very* low heat, stirring constantly until soup is thickened. Be careful not to boil or eggs will curdle.

Makes 6 servings.

This recipe is good cold and will last in the refrigerator for 4 days.

7.6 GRAMS PER SERVING

Tomato Soup

1 **quart canned tomatoes**	1 **packet sugar substitute**
2 **cups water**	1 **teaspoon salt**
3 **cloves**	2 **tablespoons butter**
¼ **cup minced onion**	1 **tablespoon arrowroot flour**

Combine first six ingredients in saucepan and simmer gently for 10 minutes. Remove from heat and strain.

Melt butter, add the flour, stirring well, and add the hot liquid slowly until no lumps appear.

Return to low heat and simmer gently for a few more minutes. Serve immediately.

Makes 4 servings.

7.4 GRAMS PER SERVING

Main Dishes

Armenian Stew

2 pounds lamb, cut into
    cubes
2 lamb shank bones
3 tablespoons olive oil
1 large onion, chopped

2 garlic cloves, minced
1 cup sliced carrots
3 medium zucchini, sliced
Salt and pepper to taste

Wash lamb, and remove any excess fat.

Heat the oil in a large pot, add the lamb, and sauté until brown.

Add onion, garlic, and enough water to cover. Simmer for 1 hour.

Add remaining ingredients; simmer for 1 hour.
Makes 4 servings.

11.3 GRAMS PER SERVING

Sole with Nut and Seed Sauce

6 fillets of sole or flounder
20 blanched almonds
¼ cup pine nuts
¼ cup sunflower seeds
2 tablespoons sesame seeds
2 cloves garlic, minced

2 tablespoons chopped
    parsley
Pinch of saffron
Seasoned salt and pepper to
    taste
6 tablespoons melted butter

Place fish in a saucepan with enough hot water to cover. Simmer a few minutes until fish flakes easily.

Place remaining ingredients in blender, stopping the blender long enough to push mixture down from sides. Blend until everything is well ground.

Drain fish, reserving water.

Gradually add some water that the fish has been cooked in to the nut mixture, to make a thick sauce. Mix well. Add melted butter. Pour over fish. Heat and serve.

Makes 6 servings.

7.1 GRAMS PER SERVING

Crabmeat with Cheese

1 **pound crabmeat, flaked and picked over**
¾ **cup chopped onion**
¼ **cup peanut oil**
2 **tablespoons curry powder**
2 **tablespoons minced parsley**
¼ **teaspoon crushed red pepper**

2 **tablespoons lemon juice**
½ **teaspoon seasoned salt**
½ **teaspoon black pepper**
¼ **teaspoon oregano**
½ **cup grated Parmesan cheese**
2 **tablespoons butter**
1 **lemon, cut into wedges**

Preheat broiler.

Sauté the onion in peanut oil until soft. Add the curry powder and cook, stirring constantly, for 1 minute.

Stir in the crabmeat, parsley, and red pepper, and sauté for 2 minutes. Add the lemon juice, salt, pepper, and oregano. Sauté for 1 minute more.

Divide the crabmeat mixture among 4 buttered scallop shells, sprinkle each serving with Parmesan cheese, and dot the tops with butter. Put the shells under the broiler for 2 to 3 minutes, or until the cheese is golden. Serve the shells with wedges of lemon.

Makes 4 servings.

9.6 GRAMS PER SERVING

Chicken Paprika

1 4-pound chicken, or 4
  pounds of chicken parts
3 tablespoons butter
1 medium onion, sliced
1 cup mushrooms, sliced
1 cup bran

¼ cup oil
½ cup chicken broth
½ cup sour cream
1½ teaspoons paprika
1 tablespoon parsley

Heat butter in a large skillet and sauté onion and mushrooms until they are golden.

Roll chicken pieces in bran.

Remove onion and mushrooms from skillet and add the oil. Sauté chicken pieces until browned. Add broth, sautéed onion, and mushrooms. Simmer 40 minutes.

Remove chicken to serving platter. Add sour cream and paprika to skillet. Heat and stir well. Do not boil. Pour sauce over chicken. Garnish with parsley.

Makes 8 servings.

8.0 GRAMS PER SERVING

Curried Chicken Avocado

2 ripe avocados
2 cooked chicken breasts,
  skinned and boned
6 tablespoons mayonnaise
2 tablespoons curry powder

½ teaspoon cumin
½ teaspoon coriander
½ pound seedless green
  grapes
Chopped walnuts

Halve avocados, remove pit, and cut meat into bite-size pieces, being careful not to break the skin. Set the avocado shells aside.

Cut chicken breasts into small pieces.

Combine avocado, chicken, mayonnaise, curry powder, cumin, coriander, and grapes. Mix well.

Fill avocado shells with the mixture and sprinkle with chopped walnuts.

Makes 4 servings.

18.0 GRAMS PER SERVING

A Gift from the Sea

1½ pounds fillet of sole or flounder
Salt and pepper to taste
½ cup Hi-Protein Soya bread crumbs (optional, page 115)

4 tablespoons butter
2 tablespoons oil
2 cloves garlic, minced
¼ cup chopped parsley
1 anchovy, mashed

Wash fillets. Sprinkle with salt and pepper. If desired, cover with bread crumbs.

Combine 2 tablespoons butter and oil in skillet. Sauté the fish to golden brown, turning once.

Remove fish to a warm platter. Place 2 tablespoons butter, garlic, parsley, and anchovy in skillet. Stir well. Sauté for 2 minutes until the garlic is golden brown. Dribble over fish fillets. Serve immediately.

Makes 4 servings.

6.0 GRAMS PER SERVING

Sautéed Fish

2 pounds fish fillets or 1 small fish
¼ cup cream
½ teaspoon seasoned salt

½ teaspoon garlic salt
1 cup Hi-Protein bread crumbs (page 115)
4 tablespoons butter

Wash and dry the fish.

Combine cream, seasoned salt, and garlic salt in a bowl. Place the bread crumbs in a dish. Dip fish in cream, then in bread crumbs.

Heat butter in a skillet without browning. Sauté fish in butter until golden brown. Serve with Parsley Butter (page 113).

Makes 4 servings.

6.9 GRAMS PER SERVING

Fried Scallops

1 pound scallops	**½ teaspoon seasoned salt**
1 cup Hi-Protein bread crumbs	**4 tablespoons butter**
	Tartar Sauce (page 235)

Drain and wash scallops.

Roll in bread crumbs and salt.

Heat butter until it foams.

Sauté scallops, turning frequently until brown on all sides, about 3 to 4 minutes.

Serve with Tartar Sauce.

Makes 2 servings.

7.0 GRAMS PER SERVING
9.3 GRAMS WITH ½ CUP SAUCE

Wok Steak 2

1 pound beef fillet or London broil, sliced thin	**½ can water chestnuts**
6 tablespoons peanut oil	**2 tablespoons sesame seeds**
1 medium onion, sliced	**2 tablespoons bottled steak sauce**
1 large zucchini, sliced thin	
½ pound snow pea pods	**¼ pound bean sprouts**
½ pound mushrooms, sliced	**3 tablespoons dark soy sauce**

Heat wok with 2 tablespoons of oil. Add vegetables, one at a time, in order of listing, allowing 1 minute cooking time between each addition. Add sesame seeds and 2 more tablespoons oil. Toss well.

Sprinkle steak with steak sauce and mix well.

Move vegetables to one side of wok. Add remaining oil in the bottom and place steak in the oil. Cook about 1 minute more.

Toss steak with vegetables. Add bean sprouts and soy sauce. Serve immediately.

Makes 8 servings.

8.0 GRAMS PER SERVING

Vitello Tonnato

3–4 pounds boneless shoulder
    or leg of veal
2 tablespoons olive oil
1 large onion, quartered
2 carrots, chopped
2 celery stalks, chopped
2 large garlic cloves, minced
1 can anchovy fillets
1 can tuna fish

1 cup dry white wine
3 sprigs parsley
Pinch thyme
½ teaspoon salt
Black pepper to taste
1 cup mayonnaise
Juice of 1 lemon
2 tablespoons capers

Heat olive oil in a large, heavy pot. Add veal and brown slightly.

Add onion, carrots, celery, garlic, anchovy fillets, tuna fish, wine, parsley, thyme, salt, and pepper. Cover pot tightly, and cook for 2 hours. Remove meat and chill.

Reduce contents of pot in half, by boiling down, and puree. Blend with mayonnaise and season with lemon juice. Chill. Serve cold. Slice veal very thin, sprinkle with capers, and serve with lemon mayonnaise.

Makes 6 servings.

7.6 GRAMS PER SERVING

Vegetables

———◆———

Eggplant Stew

5 tablespoons butter
1 pound eggplant
1 teaspoon lemon juice
⅓ cup chopped celery
¼ cup chopped onions
½ cup chopped green peppers
¼ cup chopped red peppers
1 clove garlic, minced

1 tablespoon salt
½ teaspoon marjoram
½ teaspoon tarragon
1 cup fresh tomatoes, skinned, seeded, and diced
¾ cup dry Vermouth
2 tablespoons chopped parsley

Heat butter in frying pan. Meanwhile, chop unpeeled eggplant into chunks and sprinkle with lemon juice. Add celery, onions, peppers, and garlic to butter until golden. Add eggplant and cook for 5 minutes more. Add seasonings, tomatoes, and Vermouth, stir well, cover and simmer for 10 minutes more. Uncover, and simmer until eggplant is just tender. Sprinkle with chopped parsley and serve.

Makes 4 servings.

14.2 GRAMS PER SERVING

218

Plaki (Armenian Marinated Beans)

1 cup northern beans	2 tablespoons chopped
4 cups water	fresh parsley
2 carrots, diced	1½ tablespoons salt
1 onion, sliced	1 teaspoon black pepper
1 stalk celery with leaves,	½ cup olive oil
chopped	1 teaspoon dill
3 cloves garlic, minced	¼ cup sesame seeds
4 tablespoons tomato sauce	Lemon wedges

Rinse beans well. Place beans and 4 cups water in a large pot, bring to a boil, and simmer for 5 minutes. Remove from heat. Cover and let them sit for 2 hours (or soak overnight in refrigerator).

Bring beans to a boil, add carrots, onion, celery, garlic, tomato sauce, parsley, salt, and pepper. Simmer partially covered for 1¾ hours. Add olive oil and dill, and simmer for 15 minutes more.

Refrigerate for a few hours (this enhances the flavor).

Serve hot, or at room temperature, with sesame seeds sprinkled on top and garnished with lemon wedges.

Makes 6 servings.

13.4 GRAMS PER SERVING

Carrots and Herbs

2 bunches very thin carrots	¼ teaspoon chopped dill
⅔ cup hot water	¼ teaspoon chopped parsley
2 teaspoons salt	¼ teaspoon savory flakes
6 tablespoons butter	

Preheat oven to 350°.

Slice carrots in half lengthwise, and place in shallow baking dish with water, salt, and butter. Sprinkle with herbs. Cover and bake for 45 minutes.

Makes 6 servings.

7.9 GRAMS PER SERVING

Cauliflower with Nuts and Seeds

1 medium cauliflower
5 tablespoons butter
½ cup slivered almonds
½ cup sunflower seeds

1 clove garlic, minced
1 cup Hi-Protein Soya bread crumbs
Salt and pepper to taste

Steam cauliflower for 20 minutes. Heat butter in a skillet, add remaining ingredients, and sauté until golden. Serve over cauliflower.

Makes 6 servings.

14.7 GRAMS PER SERVING

Wok Celery Side Dish Len

1 tablespoon peanut oil
4 stalks celery, diced
1 onion, sliced

2 tablespoons sesame seeds
1 tablespoon wheat germ

Heat oil in the wok. Add celery and onion. Cook for 3 minutes. Stir in sesame seeds and wheat germ and serve.

Makes 2 servings.

12.9 GRAMS PER SERVING

Pungent Cabbage

3 tablespoons safflower oil
2 large carrots, grated
3 large tomatoes, peeled and chopped
2 tablespoons arrowroot flour
1 cup chicken stock

3 tablespoons soy sauce
1 tablespoon honey
1 tablespoon molasses
1 tablespoon lemon juice
1 tablespoon wine vinegar
1 large cabbage
2 tablespoons sherry

Heat 1 tablespoon oil in heavy skillet and add the carrots and tomatoes. Fry for 3 minutes, stirring constantly.

Dissolve arrowroot in 2 tablespoons cold water, and add chicken stock, soy sauce, honey, molasses, lemon juice, and vinegar. Add to the vegetable mixture and bring to a boil, stirring constantly, until it thickens. Remove from heat and keep warm.

Shred the cabbage. Heat the remaining 2 tablespoons of oil in a large skillet and fry cabbage for 5 minutes, stirring continuously. Add the sherry and cook for 2 more minutes.

Place cabbage on a serving dish and pour the warm sauce over it.

Makes 6 servings.

14.2 GRAMS PER SERVING

Winter Squash

1 winter squash
2 packets sugar substitute
1 teaspoon cinnamon

½ cup butter
1 teaspoon salt

Preheat oven to 300°.

Peel squash and dice. Place in water to cover and cover pot. Cook 20 minutes or until soft. Drain.

Add sugar substitute, cinnamon, butter, and salt. Mash with fork or puree with food mill or food processor.

Bake in a greased ovenproof dish for 35 minutes.

Makes 4 servings.

8.1 GRAMS PER SERVING

Broccoli Caraway Soufflé

5 eggs, separated
1 cup grated Caraway cheese
¾ cup heavy cream
1 10-ounce package frozen chopped broccoli,

slightly thawed (or fresh, steamed 3 minutes and chopped)
¼ teaspoon salt
Pinch pepper

Preheat oven to 350°.

Place all ingredients except egg whites in blender or food processor. Puree until smooth.

Beat egg whites until stiff peaks form. Fold into broccoli mixture. Pour into greased soufflé dish.

Bake for 1 hour and serve immediately.

Makes 4 servings.

7.3 GRAMS PER SERVING

Broccoli Casserole

1 bunch broccoli
1 cup sour cream
½ cup water
½ cup shredded American cheese
1 tablespoon lemon juice

1 tablespoon basil
3 tablespoons toasted slivered almonds
3 tablespoons natural sunflower seeds
½ teaspoon seasoned salt

Preheat broiler.

Rinse broccoli well, discard outer leaves, cut off tough ends, and split heavy stalks lengthwise.

In a saucepan bring ½ inch of water to boil. Place broccoli in boiling water, reduce heat, simmer tightly covered about 9 minutes.

Combine the remaining ingredients.

Place broccoli in baking dish. Spoon sauce over and place under broiler until cheese begins to melt.

Serve with plain broiled meat, chicken, or fish.

Makes 6 servings.

9.6 GRAMS PER SERVING

Broccoli with Sharp Sauce

1 bunch fresh broccoli, chopped, or 2 packages frozen
½ teaspoon salt
1 packet sugar substitute
½ teaspoon paprika

2 tablespoons lemon juice
2 tablespoons butter, melted
1½ teaspoons prepared white horseradish
1 tablespoon dry white wine

Preheat oven to 350°.

Cook broccoli in lightly salted boiling water until slightly tender. Drain well.

Blend remaining ingredients together until smooth. Place broccoli in ovenproof serving dish and cover with sauce. Bake for 5-10 minutes to heat through.

Makes 4 servings.

8.6 GRAMS PER SERVING

Baked Eggplant with Cheese

1 medium eggplant
1 cup grated Parmesan
    cheese
1 medium onion, minced
1 egg

2 teaspoons parsley
Salt and pepper to taste
3 tablespoons olive oil
1 large tomato, sliced

Preheat oven to 300°.

Wash eggplant and cut into ¼-inch slices.

Combine cheese, onion, egg, parsley, salt, and pepper.

Place slices of eggplant in a well-oiled baking dish. Dribble on olive oil, and top with tomato slices.

Bake for 1 hour.

Makes 4 servings.

8.4 GRAMS PER SERVING

Special Special Spinach

3 tablespoons butter
1 small onion. sliced
¼ pound mushrooms, sliced
1 pound spinach, cooked,
    drained, and chopped

¼ cup grated Parmesan
    cheese
½ teaspoon seasoned salt
¼ cup sour cream
1 tablespoon minced parsley

Preheat oven to 375°.

Melt butter in a skillet. Add onion and mushrooms and sauté until golden.

Add spinach, Parmesan cheese, and salt. Mix well.

Place in a small buttered casserole dish. Top with sour cream and sprinkle with parsley.

Bake for 20 minutes. Serve with plain broiled meat, chicken, or fish.

Makes 4 servings.

9.1 GRAMS PER SERVING

Stuffed Tomatoes

6 medium tomatoes
1 tablespoon butter
1 onion, diced
12 fresh mushrooms (stems removed), sliced
1 teaspoon dried tarragon leaves

1 teaspoon salt
2 eggs
½ cup yogurt
½ teaspoon lemon juice
¼ teaspoon black pepper

Preheat oven to 400°.

Wash tomatoes. Cut a thin, horizontal slice in stem end of each tomato. Carefully hollow out tomatoes, reserving pulp for another use.

Turn tomatoes over and allow to drain. Place them upright in shallow baking dish.

Sauté onion in hot butter. Add mushrooms, tarragon, and salt. Cook, stirring, for 5 minutes. Beat eggs, yogurt, lemon juice, and pepper together. Stir into mushroom mixture and fill tomatoes. Bake for 20 minutes.

Makes 6 servings.

7.0 GRAMS PER SERVING

Salads

———◆———

Healthy Cottage Cheese Salad

1 pound cottage cheese
1 cup sour cream
1 green pepper, diced
1 cucumber, diced
6 scallions, minced
1 tablespoon dill
1 tablespoon tarragon

1 tablespoon basil
½ cup pumpkin seeds
¼ cup lecithin granules
1 teaspoon salt
Pepper to taste
Mixed greens

Combine all ingredients except the mixed greens. Blend well.
Serve on any salad greens, with or without a dressing.
Makes 6 servings.

11.6 GRAMS PER SERVING

Summer Salad 1

½ pound string beans,
     cleaned and cut into
     2-inch lengths
1 bunch asparagus, cleaned
     and cut into 2-inch
     lengths
1 head Boston lettuce,
     cleaned and shredded
3 tomatoes, coarsely
     chopped
2 green peppers, seeded and
     coarsely chopped

4 tablespoons chopped
     watercress
4 tablespoons chopped
     parsley
2 tablespoons fresh dill, or 1
     tablespoon dried dill
2 tablespoons prepared
     mustard
¼ cup vinegar
¼ cup olive oil
½ packet sugar substitute

Steam string beans and asparagus for 5 minutes. Allow to
cool. Place in a salad bowl and add lettuce, tomatoes, green
peppers, watercress, parsley, and dill. Mix well.

Mix mustard with vinegar, add olive oil and sugar substitute. Mix well and pour over vegetables.

Makes 8 servings.

18.0 GRAMS PER SERVING

Summer Salad 2

To the above recipe add:

1 can tuna, drained
12 black olives, pitted and
     sliced

1 can pimiento, chopped

Makes 6 servings.

19.6 GRAMS PER SERVING

Continental Salad

1 cup thinly sliced snow pea
    pods
1 medium zucchini, thinly
    sliced and finely chopped
1 cup finely chopped broc-
    coli flowerets

1 cup thinly sliced mush-
    rooms
1 cup cherry tomatoes
¼ cup pine nuts

Combine all ingredients and serve with salad dressing of your
choice.
    Makes 4 servings.

12.0 GRAMS PER SERVING

Cold Green Bean Salad with Nuts

1 pound cooked green beans
½ cup French Dressing
1 small onion, grated

½ cup slivered almonds
¼ cup sesame seeds

Drain beans well. Add dressing and onion. Chill thoroughly.
    Sprinkle with almonds and sesame seeds. Serve on lettuce
leaves if desired.
    Makes 4 servings.

15.9 GRAMS PER SERVING

Bean Sprout Salad

1 cup bean sprouts
1 cup diced zucchini
1 tomato, diced

1 carrot, grated
½ cup sesame seeds
Avocado Dressing (page 234)

Toss all ingredients together except dressing.

Pour dressing over salad before serving. Toss again.

Makes 4 servings.

15.0 GRAMS PER SERVING

Crisp Chinese Salad

1 cup alfalfa sprouts
1 cup shredded lettuce
½ cup diced green pepper
½ cup diced green onions
¼ cup diced celery

1 diced cucumber
1 cup cooked peas
¼ cup bran
Thousand Island Dressing
    (page 234)

Toss ingredients together in a salad bowl. Add dressing.

Makes 8 servings.

10.8 GRAMS PER SERVING

Greek Salad

1 large cucumber, pared and
    cubed
1 large tomato, cubed
8 radishes, sliced
½ cup pitted black olives
4 scallions, sliced
¼ pound Feta cheese,
    crumbled

3 tablespoons wine vinegar
6 tablespoons olive oil
½ teaspoon oregano
¼ teaspoon black pepper
½ head romaine or iceberg
    lettuce

Combine cucumber, tomato, radishes, olives, scallions, and cheese in a bowl.

Mix wine vinegar, olive oil, oregano, and pepper together. Pour over vegetables, and toss.

Cover and refrigerate for 1 hour.

Tear lettuce in bite-sized pieces.
Add vegetables with dressing, and toss.
Makes 2 servings.

13.0 GRAMS PER SERVING

Salade Niçoise

2 teaspoons Dijon mustard
2 tablespoons wine vinegar
1½ teaspoons salt
2 cloves garlic, minced
6 tablespoons peanut or vegetable oil
6 tablespoons olive oil
Freshly ground black pepper
1 teaspoon chopped fresh thyme, or ½ teaspoon dried
2 pounds green beans
2 green peppers
4 celery stalks

1 pint cherry tomatoes
3 7-ounce cans tuna
1 2-ounce can flat anchovies
10 stuffed green olives
10 black olives
2 small or 1 large red onion
2 tablespoons chopped fresh basil, or 1 teaspoon dried
⅓ cup finely chopped fresh parsley
¼ cup finely chopped scallions
6 hard-boiled eggs, quartered

Combine the mustard, vinegar, salt, garlic, peanut and olive oil, pepper, and thyme in a bowl. Beat with a fork until well blended. Set aside.

Pick over the beans and break them into 1½-inch lengths. Place them in a saucepan and cook, in salted water to cover, until tender but crisp. Drain and run under cold water. Drain in a colander. Set aside.

Remove the cores, seeds and white membranes from the green peppers. Cut the peppers in thin rounds. Set aside.

Trim the celery stalks and cut crosswise into thin slices. Set aside.

Bring a quart of water to a boil. Drop in the cherry tomatoes and let stand for exactly 15 seconds. Drain immediately. Pull off the tomato skins with a paring knife. Set tomatoes aside.

Use a large salad bowl and make a more or less symmetrical pattern of the green beans, peppers, celery, and tomatoes. Flake the tuna fish and add to bowl. Arrange anchovies on top and scatter olives over all.

Peel the onions and cut them into thin, almost transparent slices. Scatter the onion rings over all. Sprinkle with basil, parsley, and scallions. Garnish with eggs.

Toss salad with dressing after garnished bowl has been presented.

Makes 12 servings.

10.6 GRAMS PER SERVING

Hearty Seafood Salad

1 cup tuna, or 1
    7-ounce can, drained
1 cup crabmeat, or 1
    7-ounce can, drained
1 cup lobster, or 1
    7-ounce can, drained
1 cup shrimp, or 1
    7-ounce can, drained
1 head lettuce, shredded
1 cup sliced celery
8 scallions, thinly sliced
1 cucumber, sliced
½ cup sliced radishes

3 hard-boiled eggs, diced
2 tomatoes, chopped
1 avocado, diced
4 tablespoons lemon juice
½ cup slivered almonds or
    chopped walnuts
¼ cup wheat germ
2 tablespoons lecithin granules
1 recipe Creamy Celery
    Seed Dressing
    (page 109)

Discard any bone or skin from seafood and cut into small chunks. Combine seafood, cover, and chill.

Combine lettuce, celery, scallions, cucumber, and radishes in a large bowl. Chill.

Add eggs, tomatoes, and avocado tossed in lemon juice to lettuce combination.

Add seafood, almonds or walnuts, wheat germ, and lecithin granules.

Toss with dressing.
Makes 10 servings.

11.8 GRAMS PER SERVING

Turkey Salad

- 1 cup diced turkey
- ½ cup diced celery
- ¼ cup finely chopped scallions

- 1 orange, finely chopped
- 1 cup seedless green grapes

Combine all ingredients and serve with Curry Dressing (page 110).
Makes 2 servings.

15.0 GRAMS PER SERVING

Broccoli Sunflower Seed Salad

- 1 small head of Boston lettuce
- 1 cup chopped raw broccoli
- 1 medium zucchini, sliced

- 3 tablespoons sunflower seeds
- 2 tablespoons lecithin
- Sour Cream Mayonnaise Dressing (page 112)

Combine all ingredients. Toss well.
Makes 4 servings.

8.5 GRAMS PER SERVING

Nutty Chicken Salad

3 cups diced and cooked
    chicken
1 cup diced celery
2 cups diced melon
½ cup heavy cream
2 tablespoons lecithin
    (optional)

1 cup Sweet Fruity
    Dressing (page 235)
½ cup toasted almonds or
    pecans
¼ cup toasted pumpkin
    seeds
½ cup coconut

Combine chicken, celery, and melon in a large bowl.

Chill.

Just before serving, whip cream and fold in lecithin and dressing.

Pour dressing over chicken mixture. Sprinkle nuts, seeds, and coconut on top and toss together gently.

Makes 8 servings.

14.7 GRAMS PER SERVING FRUITY DRESSING

Dressings, Sauces, and Jams

———◆———

Avocado Dressing

4 tablespoons tarragon vinegar
2 tablespoons sour cream
1 teaspoon wheat germ
1 teaspoon wheat germ

½ teaspoon dry mustard
1 teaspoon Dijon mustard
¼ teaspoon garlic powder
1 egg
1 small avocado, diced

Combine all ingredients in screw-top jar. Shake well. Refrigerate.

TOTAL GRAMS 9.4

Thousand Island Dressing

4 tablespoons vinegar
2 tablespoons olive oil
6 tablespoons safflower oil
2 tablespoons mayonnaise
1 tablespoon lemon juice
4 tablespoons tomato juice

2 tablespoons chopped green
   olives
2 tablespoons sunflower
   seeds
1 packet sugar substitute
1 egg

Place all ingredients in a screw-top jar. Shake well. Refrigerate.

TOTAL GRAMS 14.0

Yogurt Dressing

8 tablespoons olive oil
12 tablespoons safflower oil
12 tablespoons tarragon vinegar
1 teaspoon seasoned salt
1 tablespoon dill

1 tablespoon tarragon
1 tablespoon Dijon mustard
½ teaspoon garlic powder
3 tablespoons yogurt
1 tablespoon liquid lecithin
1 packet sugar substitute

Place all ingredients in a screw-top jar. Shake well. Refrigerate.

Makes 2½ cups.

TOTAL GRAMS 11.5

Sweet Fruity Dressing

½ cup heavy cream
2 tablespoons lemon juice

1½ tablespoons Grand Marnier

In a medium-size bowl whip the cream until it piles softly.

Add lemon juice and liqueur. Beat a few seconds more until blended.

Serve on fruit, tablespoon.

TOTAL GRAMS 25.2

Tartar Sauce

¾ cup sour cream or mayonnaise
1 tablespoon finely chopped pickle
1 tablespoon finely chopped onion

1 tablespoon finely chopped olives
1 teaspoon tarragon
1 teaspoon parsley

Combine all ingredients. Mix well.

Store in covered jar in refrigerator.

Makes 1 cup.

9.9 GRAMS WITH MAYONNAISE
9.3 GRAMS WITH SOUR CREAM

Pasta Sauce, Red

3 tablespoons olive oil
2 pounds chopped beef
1 pound Italian sweet
    sausage
1 teaspoon seasoned salt
½ onion, finely chopped

2 cloves garlic, minced
32 ounces tomato juice
2 8-ounce cans tomato sauce
4 cups water
2 bay leaves

Pour olive oil into a heavy skillet and add chopped meat.

Place the sausage in a separate skillet and let it brown slowly. Remove from pan and cut into pieces.

Season meat with salt. Add onion and garlic to the skillet with the chopped meat and allow to brown.

Heat tomato juice, tomato sauce, and water in a large pot. Add bay leaves, cooked sausage, and browned meat mixture. Allow to simmer for 2½ hours.

Makes 6 cups.

TOTAL GRAMS 83.8

All-Purpose Garnish

1 tablespoon walnuts
1 tablespoon sesame seeds
1 tablespoon almonds
1 tablespoon sunflower seeds
1 tablespoon pumpkin seeds

1 teaspoon caraway seeds
1 teaspoon chives
½ teaspoon seasoned salt
⅛ teaspoon cayenne pepper

Combine all ingredients in a wooden chopping bowl. Chop fine.

TOTAL GRAMS 13.1

Blueberries and Wine Sauce

1 pint fresh blueberries,
    thawed if frozen
½ cup Burgundy wine

1 packet sugar substitute,
    brown if possible
2 tablespoons cognac

Combine blueberries with wine and sugar substitute and chill for an hour.

Place in saucepan and cook on very low flame until berries boil (about 5 minutes). Stir often.

Pour cognac over berries and ignite. Serve flaming over any plain cake or custard.

Makes 8 servings.

8.1 GRAMS PER SERVING

Blueberry Jam

1 cup blueberries at room
    temperature
1 tablespoon arrowroot
1 envelope unflavored
    gelatin

2 tablespoons cold water
2 tablespoons hot water
3 packets sugar substitute

Mix blueberries with arrowroot.

Dissolve gelatin in cold water for 5 minutes. Add hot water and stir thoroughly. Combine with blueberry mixture in saucepan and heat to boiling, stirring constantly. Boil for 2 minutes. Remove from heat. Add sugar substitute. Refrigerate.

Makes ¾ cup.

TOTAL GRAMS 39.4

Desserts

Sweet Melon

½ cup halved strawberries   4 tablespoons Anisette
½ cubed cantaloupe

Combine strawberries and melon in a bowl.
  Pour in Anisette and stir well. Cover and refrigerate for 1 hour.
  Makes 4 servings.

6.0 GRAMS PER SERVING

Anisette Dreams

½ honeydew melon   2 tablespoons Anisette

Cut melon in large cubes or balls. Place in a bowl, sprinkle with Anisette. Chill.
  Makes 5 servings.

TOTAL GRAMS 29.1
5.8 GRAMS PER SERVING

Coconut Anisette Dreams

Follow directions in preceding recipe and then roll melon in
½ cup unsweetened coconut.
Makes 5 servings.

TOTAL GRAMS 32.1
6.4 GRAMS PER SERVING

Strawberry Sherbet

1 cup heavy cream	½ teaspoon strawberry
1 tablespoon lemon juice	extract
6 packets sugar substitute	1 cup strawberries, fresh or
2 tablespoons Strawberry	frozen
liqueur	1¼ cups crushed ice
1 teaspoon vanilla	

Blend all ingredients except ice. Add ice and blend until
thickened. Serve immediately.
Makes 4 servings.

8.2 GRAMS PER SERVING

Strawberry Cheese Pudding

1 pint strawberries, sliced	1 teaspoon cinnamon
3 tablespoons Strawberry	½ teaspoon nutmeg
liqueur	¼ teaspoon ground cloves
2 cups cottage cheese	½ cup chopped walnuts
4 packets sugar substitute	2 packets brown sugar sub-
5 eggs	stitute
¼ cup sour cream	

Preheat oven to 325°.

Soak strawberries in liqueur for 1 hour. Drain and reserve liquid.

Blend cottage cheese, sugar substitute, and eggs to a smooth puree. Pour into a greased casserole dish. Arrange strawberries on top.

Stir remaining marinade into sour cream, cinnamon, nutmeg, cloves, nuts, and brown sugar substitute. Spoon over strawberries. Bake for 40 minutes. Serve hot.

Makes 6 servings.

12.1 GRAMS PER SERVING

Peppermint Raspberry Flip

½ cup raspberries   1 cup yogurt
¼ teaspoon peppermint   Fresh mint leaves
    extract

Place raspberries in a small bowl. Add peppermint extract and mix well.

Add yogurt and mix well again.

Place in dessert glasses and garnish with mint leaves. Chill.
Makes 3 servings.

7.0 GRAMS PER SERVING

Strawberries with Raspberry and Nut Topping

1 cup frozen or fresh rasp-   2 cups frozen or fresh straw-
    berries   berries, cleaned, hulled,
4 tablespoons Kirschwasser   and halved
    or Blackberry liqueur   1 teaspoon chopped nuts
2 teaspoons lemon juice

Thaw and drain raspberries, if frozen.

Place in a blender and puree.

Stir in liqueur and lemon juice. Refrigerate for at least 1 hour.

To serve, place strawberries in dessert dish, spoon raspberry puree on top, and sprinkle with nuts.

Makes 6 servings.

7.2 GRAMS PER SERVING

Strawberry Ice Cream

1 pint strawberries	6 packets sugar substitute
1½ teaspoons gelatin	1½ teaspoons vanilla extract
1½ cups heavy cream	

Place strawberries in blender and blend until pureed.

Soften gelatin in 2 tablespoons cold water.

Heat to scalding ½ cup cream over low heat. Add sugar substitute and vanilla extract; stir to dissolve. Add gelatin. Cool by placing pan in cold water. Add remaining cream and strawberries. Blend well.

Pour mixture into freezer trays, cover with transparent wrap, and freeze until firm. Or pour into your ice cream maker.

If in freezer for more than 6 hours before serving, allow to stand at room temperature for 15 minutes.

Makes 6 servings.

7.5 GRAMS PER SERVING

Uncooked Cottage Cheese Pudding

½ cup cream
3 egg yolks
4 tablespoons honey
2 cups cottage cheese
4 tablespoons butter
Grated rind of 1 lemon

1 tablespoon Grand Marnier
    liqueur or 1 teaspoon
    vanilla
Sprinkle of cinnamon
¼ cup chopped walnuts

Whip cream with a rotary beater in a large bowl. Add egg yolks and honey and beat again. Add cottage cheese, ½ cup at a time, beating well after each addition.

Add butter, lemon rind, and liqueur or vanilla. Beat well. Place in 5 dessert bowls and sprinkle with cinnamon and walnuts. Chill.

Makes 5 servings.

15.4 GRAMS PER SERVING

Pumpkin Custard

6 packets sugar substitute
1 teaspoon salt
½ teaspoon cinnamon
2 cups canned pumpkin

2 eggs, beaten
¾ cup heavy cream
¼ cup water

Preheat oven to 400°.

Mix sugar substitute, salt, and cinnamon. Add pumpkin to mixture and blend thoroughly. Gradually add eggs, cream, and water. Stir until smooth.

Spray individual custard cups with grease substitute and pour custard mixture into them. Sit cups in a shallow baking pan in oven with about 1 inch of water in the pan. Bake for 10 minutes at 400°, then reduce heat to 350° and continue baking for 30 minutes, or until a knife blade inserted into the center of custard comes out clean.

Makes 4 servings.

10.5 GRAMS PER SERVING

Custard Cream Filling

1 teaspoon gelatin
1 tablespoon cold water
3 egg yolks
2 tablespoons fructose
1 tablespoon liqueur
   (any flavor)

1 cup heavy cream
1 teaspoon vanilla,
   almond, orange, or
   lemon extract

Dissolve gelatin in cold water.

Whisk egg yolks and fructose in top of double boiler until thickened. Remove from heat. Add gelatin and liqueur and whisk until smooth. Cool.

Whip cream and extract together until soft peaks form. Fold cream into thickening egg mixture. Chill.

Makes 1¼ cups.

TOTAL GRAMS 34.0

Chocolate Frosting

1 pint heavy cream
2 tablespoons chocolate
   extract

2 packets sugar substitute
¼ packet Alba 77

Beat heavy cream, chocolate extract, sugar substitute, and Alba 77 until the cream whips. Spread between layers of cake and on top. Refrigerate.

TOTAL GRAMS 20.8

Pie Crust 2

1 cup soya flour
Pinch nutmeg
Pinch cinnamon
1 packet sugar substitute
½ cup ground blanched
   almonds

1 hard-boiled egg yolk,
   mashed
⅓ cup butter, chilled
1 raw egg yolk
½ teaspoon vanilla

Preheat oven to 400°.

Stir first 5 ingredients together. Add egg yolk. Stir thoroughly. Cut in butter. Work into dry ingredients well. Add raw egg yolk and vanilla. Stir thoroughly.

Cover with waxed paper and refrigerate for 1 hour.

Place in pie pan by tablespoons, patting sides and bottom with back of spoon. Use fork tines to decorate edges of pie crust and to prick holes in bottom and sides of crust.

Arrange empty disposable pie plate over pie (to keep crust from puffing). Bake for 30 minutes until solid and brown around edges. Remove second pan, cover edges with foil, and allow center to brown thoroughly. Cool.

TOTAL GRAMS 41.1

Pie Crust 3

1 cup soya flour
½ cup ground almonds
2 packets sugar substitute

Pinch cinnamon
⅓ cup butter, chilled

Preheat oven to 400°.

Stir first 4 ingredients together. Cut in butter. Work into dry ingredients well.

Cover with waxed paper and refrigerate for 1 hour.

Place in pie pan by tablespoons, patting sides and bottom with back of spoon. Use fork tines to decorate edges of pie crust and to prick holes in bottom and sides of crust.

Arrange empty disposable pie plate over pie (to keep crust from puffing). Bake for 30 minutes until solid and brown around edges. Remove second pan, cover edges with foil, and allow center to brown thoroughly. Cool.

TOTAL GRAMS 36.0

Lemon Chiffon Pie

3 egg yolks
1½ cups water
2 packets sugar substitute
1 package diet lemon gelatin
2 tablespoons lemon juice
1 teaspoon lemon extract

½ teaspoon grated lemon rind
3 egg whites
⅛ teaspoon salt
Pie Crust 3, baked (page 244)

Combine egg yolks, 1 cup water, and sugar substitute in saucepan. Simmer, stirring constantly, until mixture begins to boil. Remove from heat, and stir in gelatin. Add remainder of water, lemon juice, lemon extract, and rind. Chill until somewhat thickened.

Beat egg whites and salt until mixture stands in stiff peaks. Stir gelatin mixture slightly, and fold in egg whites. Pour into prepared pie crust. Chill until firm.

Makes 8 servings.

7.2 GRAMS PER SERVING

Popcorn Balls

4 cups popped corn
2 cups granola
1 cup nuts, whole or ground
1 cup honey

¼ cup water
2 teaspoons vanilla
½ cup wheat germ (optional)

Place popcorn, granola, and nuts in a large bowl. Set aside.

Heat honey and water in a small pot. When it starts to boil, turn to simmer, stirring constantly. Drop a few drops into cold water; when it forms a soft ball, it is done.

Stir in vanilla, pour over popcorn mixture. Mix well.

Wet hands with water for easier handling. Form popcorn into balls about 2 inches in diameter.

Makes 20 balls.

3.1 GRAMS PER BALL

Oatmeal Carob Nut Candy

½ cup ground sesame seeds
¼ cup ground sunflower
    seeds
1 cup rolled oatmeal
⅓ cup soy flakes

½ cup honey
1 cup chopped walnuts
2 teaspoons vanilla
⅓ cup carob

Combine all ingredients except carob and mix well. Shape into small balls and roll in carob.

Refrigerate or freeze.

Makes 60 candy balls.

5.4 GRAMS PER CANDY BALL

Frozen Peanut Candies

½ cup unsalted peanuts,
   chopped
¾ cup peanut butter

1 cup heavy cream
2 packets sugar substitute
½ cup toasted sesame seeds

Combine all ingredients. Press into shallow rectangular pan. Cut 2-inch squares with the point of a knife. Freeze. Separate as cut and serve frozen.

Makes 18 candies.

4.5 GRAMS PER CANDY

Chocolate Fudge

2 packages diet chocolate
   pudding
8 packets sugar substitute
   (brown if possible)
1 cup heavy cream
1 teaspoon vanilla

2 tablespoons Crème de
   Cacao
1 12-ounce jar chunky
   peanut butter
1 cup chopped walnuts
1 cup unprocessed bran

Combine pudding, sugar substitute, cream, vanilla, and Crème de Cacao in a saucepan over low heat. Stir until smooth. Add peanut butter and stir until melted and well mixed. Gradually add walnuts and bran, and stir until well blended.

Spray 8-inch square baking pan with grease substitute and pour fudge mixture into pan.

Freeze until solid. Cut fudge into squares.

Makes 24 squares.

6.1 GRAMS PER SQUARE

Sesame Seed Candy

1 cup ground sesame seeds	**1 teaspoon vanilla**
3 tablespoons oil	**½ teaspoon rum flavoring**
2 tablespoons honey	

Combine all ingredients in a bowl. Mix well.

Knead with your hands for 2 minutes, then roll into a log ¾ inch thick. Slice into small logs about 2 inches long.

Refrigerate before serving.

Makes 24 candies.

2.6 GRAMS PER CANDY

Carob Sesame Seed Candy

Follow preceding recipe, adding 1 tablespoon carob to ingredients.

Makes 24 candies.

2.9 GRAMS PER CANDY

Peanut Butter Sesame Seed Candy

Follow preceding recipe, adding 1 tablespoon peanut butter. Roll in ⅓ cup unsweetened coconut.

Makes 24 candies.

2.8 GRAMS PER CANDY

Sesame Seed and Nut Candy

½ cup sesame meal
½ cup chopped almonds
2 tablespoons oil

2 tablespoons honey
1 teaspoon vanilla
½ teaspoon almond extract

Combine all ingredients in a bowl. Mix well.
Follow directions for Sesame Seed Candy.
Makes 24 candies.

2.6 GRAMS PER CANDY

Beverages

———◆———

Peanut Shake

3½ cups water
½ cup cream
1 cup peanuts

2 tablespoons honey
1 teaspoon vanilla
2 tablespoons brewer's yeast

Place all ingredients in a blender. Blend well. Chill.
Makes 6 servings.

12.3 GRAMS PER SERVING

Hot Mint Chocolate Nog

1 cup Pelican Punch herbal tea (available in specialty and health food stores
2 teaspoons artificially sweetened chocolate syrup

1 teaspoon chocolate extract
1 packet sugar substitute
1 egg
2 tablespoons heavy cream
1 heaping teaspoon brewer's yeast

Place all ingredients in blender. Blend well.
Makes 1 serving.

TOTAL GRAMS 4.4

Mocha Bran Shake

2 cups water
1 cup cream
8 ice cubes
3 tablespoons bran
1 tablespoon Pero (instant coffee)

2 tablespoons unsulfured molasses
¼ cup blanched almonds
1 teaspoon vanilla

Combine all ingredients in a blender. Blend well.
Serve immediately.

Makes 2 servings.

16.1 GRAMS PER SERVING

Herbal Bloody Mary

1 teaspoon Capsicum herb tea (available in specialty and health food stores)

½ cup boiling water
32 ounces tomato juice
1 tablespoon wheat germ
¼ cup vodka (optional)

Place tea in boiling water. Allow to steep for 6 minutes.
Strain tea, discard herbs, and add liquid to tomato juice. Mix
in wheat germ and vodka.
Makes 8 4-ounce servings.

5.1 GRAMS PER SERVING

Nut-Bran Shake

2 cups water
1 cup cream
6 ice cubes
3 tablespoons bran

2 tablespoons unsulfured
   molasses
¼ cup blanched almonds
1 teaspoon almond extract

Place all ingredients in a blender. Blend well. Serve immediately.

Makes 4 servings.

9.3 GRAMS PER SERVING

CHARTS

VITAMIN CHART

VITAMIN	FOOD SOURCES
A (Carotene)	Eggs Green, leafy vegetables Liver Whole milk and milk products Yellow fruits and vegetables
B Complex: B_1 (Thiamine)	Brewer's yeast Brown rice Cantaloupe Egg yolks Endive Grapefruit Green lima beans Legumes Meat, fish, and poultry Milk Molasses Nuts Organ meats Potatoes

VITAMIN	FOOD SOURCES
	Tomatoes
	Whole grains
B₂	
(Riboflavin)	Beets
	Brewer's yeast
	Carrots
	Cottage cheese
	Crabmeat
	Egg yolks
	Fish
	Green leafy vegetables
	Legumes
	Milk
	Molasses
	Nuts
	Organ meats
	Oysters
	Peaches
	Pears
	Prunes
	Tomatoes
	Whole grains
B₃	Brewer's yeast
(Niacin)	Fish
	Lean meats
	Liver
	Peanuts
	Poultry
	Rice bran
B₆	RAW:
	Avocados

VITAMIN	FOOD SOURCES
	Bananas
	Cabbage
	Carrots
	Green, leafy vegetables
	Green peppers
	Peanuts
	Pecans
	COOKED:
	Legumes
	Meats
	Organ meats
	Whole grains
B_{12} (Cyanocobalamin) and Folic Acid	Animal protein is almost the only source in which it occurs in sufficient amounts: Dairy products: milk, milk powder, eggs, and cheese Fish Kidney Liver Muscle meats
B_{13} (Orotic Acid)	Liquid whey Root vegetables
BIOTIN	Egg yolks Legumes Liver Sardines Unpolished rice Whole grains

VITAMIN	FOOD SOURCES
INOSITOL	Brewer's yeast
	Citrus fruits
	Meat
	Milk
	Molasses
	Nuts
	Vegetables
	Whole grains
PABA (Para-Aminobenzoic Acid)	Brewer's yeast
	Eggs
	Liver
	Milk
	Molasses
	Wheat germ
	Whole rice cereals
	Whole wheat
	Yogurt
B_{15} (Pangamic Acid)	Brewer's yeast
	Brown rice
	Rare steak
	Sunflower, pumpkin, and sesame seeds
B_{17} (laetrile)	Whole kernels of apricots, apples, cherries, peaches, and plums
C Complex	Alfalfa, seeds and sprouts
	Avocado
	Banana (for children)
	Broccoli
	Brussels sprouts

                               Cabbage, raw
                               Cantaloupe
                               Cauliflower

Cabbage, raw
Cantaloupe
Cauliflower
Citrus fruit
Currants
Green pepper
Kale
Kohlrabi
Papaya
Parsnips
Peppers
Potatoes
Raspberries
Rose hips
Strawberries
Tomatoes
Watercress

E

Eggs
Green, leafy vegetables
Molasses
Organ meats
Sweet potatoes
Vegetable oils:
    Corn
    Linseed
    Olive
    Poppy seed
    Tung

F

Butter
Sunflower seeds
Vegetable oils

K

Cauliflower
Egg yolks

VITAMIN	FOOD SOURCES
	Green, leafy vegetables
	Molasses
	Safflower oil
	Soy beans

METRIC CHARTS

Metric Quantities of a Measuring Cup

Metric Cup	Volume (Liquids)	Volume (Solids)	Powder (Flour)	Granular (Sugar)	Grain (Rice)
1	250 ml.	200 g.	140 g.	190 g.	150 g.
3/4	188 ml.	150 g.	105 g.	143 g.	113 g.
2/3	167 ml.	133 g.	93 g.	127 g.	100 g.
1/2	125 ml.	100 g.	70 g.	95 g.	75 g.
1/3	83 ml.	67 g.	47 g.	63 g.	50 g.
1/4	31 ml.	25 g.	18 g.	24 g.	19 g.

The Measuring Cup:

The milliliter replaces the ounce when used in liquid equivalents (volume).

The gram replaces the ounce when used in weight equivalents (mass).

When you know:	You can find:	If you multiply by:
Ounces	Milliliters	30
Milliliters	Ounces	0.03
Ounce	Gram	28
Gram	Ounce	0.04

Weight (Mass)—Kilograms will replace pounds:

When you know:	You can find:	If you multiply by:
Pounds	Kilograms	0.45
Kilograms	Pounds	2.2
Ounces	Grams	28
Grams	Ounces	0.035

1 Teaspoon	=	5 milliliters
1 Tablespoon	=	15 milliliters
1 Gram	=	1/28 ounce

Metric Use of the Oven:

300° Fahrenheit	Slow	150° Celsius
325° Fahrenheit	Slow	160° Celsius
350° Fahrenheit	Moderate	175° Celsius
375° Fahrenheit	Moderate	190° Celsius
400° Fahrenheit	Hot	200° Celsius
425° Fahrenheit	Hot	220° Celsius

LIQUID VOLUME—Liters replace pints, quarts, and gallons.

When you know:	You can find:	If you multiply by:
Pints	Liters	0.47
Quarts	Liters	0.95
Gallons	Liters	3.8
Liters	Pints	2.1
Liters	Quarts	1.06
Liters	Gallons	0.26

5 liters	=	1.30 gallons
5 gallons	=	19 liters
20 liters	=	21 quarts
20 quarts	=	19 liters
10 pints	=	4.7 liters
4.7 liters	=	9.9 pints

Metrics According to Ingredients

	BUTTER U.S.	Metric	FLOUR U.S.	Metric	SUGAR U.S.	Metric
Full Cup	16 (tbsp.)	220 (grams)	16 (tbsp.)	144 (grams)	10 (tbsp.)	229 (grams)
3/4 Cup	12 (tbsp.)	172 (grams)	12 (tbsp.)	108 (grams)	12 (tbsp.)	172 (grams)
1/2 Cup	8 (tbsp.)	114 (grams)	8 (tbsp.)	72 (grams)	8 (tbsp.)	114 (grams)
1/3 Cup	5+ (tbsp.)	78 (grams)	5+ (tbsp.)	46 (grams)	5+ (tbsp.)	76 (grams)
1/4 Cup	4 (tbsp.)	57 (grams)	4 (tbsp.)	36 (grams)	4 (tbsp.)	57 (grams)

	BUTTER	FLOUR	SUGAR
One tablespoon	15.0 grams	9.0 grams	15.0 grams
One teaspoon	5.0 grams	3.0 grams	5.0 grams

Index